# Detox of Your Thyroid

### Karen L. Pringle

# THE MEDICAL LEGAL DISCLAIMER

I have presented information in this book which is based entirely upon detoxification, diet and lifestyle as it relates to helping you with your own health and especially, improving the health of your thyroid gland.

This book is a way to memorialize the ways I used to help people find success on their healing journey, partnership based work that I have done in my physical business as well as with clients all over the world virtually, in individual consultations.

I am *required* to inform you:

That, any treatments, supplements, detoxification or healing should you choose to do so, should be done **only** after you have consulted with a doctor and received **approval**.

Many people feel very strongly that you should have "proper" laboratory and clinical testing and direct supervision through any healing process you decide to do for yourself.

I have therefore, written this book for informational and educational purposes only. It is not intended to be used as medical advice nor replace your doctor.

ISBN: 0-9992994-0-9
ISBN-13: 978-0-9992994-0-1

# DEDICATION

Zahwa, my Son, I love you so much-this is my life's work, and I want you to know we can improve our lives so dramatically with daily habits that truly bring success!

My Grandmothers, Olive & Etna, you are both with me always; you both showed me the ways of old and each of you suffered from thyroid imbalance in your own ways which caused me to become determined. I observed the multigenerational manifestations of thyroid afflictions throughout our family, and the families of 100s of clients so that each could learn from the symbolic roadmap from multiple perspectives: Mind Body, diet, lifestyle, environment, and more!

Anthony, I appreciate the administrative assistance and encouragement-you have truly become family. I am so thankful for the opportunity to bring this fruit!

I want to give thanks to my cousin, Nancy Jobe, who gave love and encouragement. Who makes the most beautiful earrings that I wear and that people always compliment.

I want to give thanks to Kim for always standing by me, Shannon for all the love and support, Lara, for the spiritual road and vision, and Deb Boucher for encouragement and support.

To you: for understanding that I have medicine that I gather and I work individually with people, but I am new to getting it into a book and giving it to you, and, at this time I do not have the budget to hire professional editing. I want you to have the medicine and be able to understand why thyroid is affecting so many of us and what to do about it. I want you to learn to become your own physician so that you can listen with your own body and heal yourself naturally.

# CONTENTS

# ACKNOWLEDGMENTS

I give thanks for the many teachers, mentors and elders and, as
Dr. Sebi himself said:

**…Whenever you go against the grain….**

Give thanks Dr. Sebi for your intelligence, which is rarely found today. Give
thanks to my grandmother Etna that knew the mind and intuition, and began expanding my awareness as a young girl beginning in 1965 so that I
became connected, naturally.

When we are a concrete thinker, and all is black or white, right or wrong,
medical doctor or quack we miss out on all the beautiful ways of life, nature
and medicine which is already here for us. If you do not have 'time' for the
stories you will never hear them.

# PREFACE

Thy Rod & Thy Staff they comfort me.  (23rd Psalm)

Your thyroid, situated along your staff (your cervical spine) communicates between Mind and Body. Everything in The Field is constantly communicating with the Self (cells).

We have an epidemic of thyroid gland imbalance today. Radioactive iodine and RF technology compromise us and, an entire way of life has been built which disables the heartbeat of humanity.

Detox & Heal Your Thyroid is a *recipe* for you to remember. I invite you to sit down to the table and share, as well as build so that we may again experience humanity.

# INTRODUCTION

In this book you will learn about how most people put toxic items in their grocery carts and take them home and that consuming these items causes you to develop and continue to have thyroid problems; I will explain how and why and you can reverse and heal yourself. Remove bromine from your life and energize yourself.

I cover detoxification, minerals, and elements like iodine and about why you should not be surprised that often, doctors do not find your thyroid imbalance on a blood test. It was even more difficult when I spoke with a doctor about thyroid imbalance causing intense anxiety and depression as well as extreme lethargy. Thyroid issues often produce **emotional and mental issues** for many people. In fact, thyroid imbalance is pandemic and epidemic right now! People in Africa are suffering from preventable thyroid imbalances like cretinism and in many other places in the world children are being born with central nervous system dysfunction that is exacerbated by the use of toxins in our everyday lives.

I worked hard on this book and I never feel done with seeking and re-search: my mind is very inquisitive and I feel and experience life very passionately. I spent thousands of hours, reading, learning, helping people heal in many ways, healing my own thyroid. I spent a lot of time in meditation, listening. A lot of time outside walking and being shown through the beauty of nature.

I began to sift quite easily through the predictable. I have seen and experienced much in life.

I settled upon the title of this book because I wanted it to represent quite simply what must be done to heal your own thyroid gland: detox and heal.

Your thyroid gland has been under attack! Radioactive Iodine, the products you eat, drink and use cause it to become swollen, inflamed, slow, fast and diseased with lumps, bumps, cysts, nodules and tumors. I guide you with step by step to write down your own plan, to observe family patterns and multigenerational issues and more.

Take the offenders out of the equation and you get better almost instantly! Participate for several months following my suggestions in the book and watch miracles happen! Not just some of the time-all of the time! And, these recommendations are also very anti-aging!

**No results? You did not stay the course**, it is that simple. Sneaking and treating with offending foods, drinks, drugs, and lifestyle habits only serves to sabotage you! Oral gratification and treats are a part of our culture and language, but if you can discipline yourself to save money, to do your chores, get up in the morning and get to work, school or your business, and keep your home relatively tidy you can easily set up a plan for yourself to do what I have in this book.

**Clients told me that they felt really awake! That they saw the world through a new lens, one that had hope and promise, because if they could feel this good, why on Earth were so many people resisting doing it?**

**Change is not comfortable for many people**, are you the type that is so hungry to take care of yourself and live that you will take time out for you? That you can read through this book, write down your plan and do it?

If you are tired and feeling unwell, low energy, overweight, anxious, and wondering if doctors can figure out what on Earth is wrong with you-why you feel so poorly? Or, perhaps you just accepted that you are going to be taking Thyroid medications for the rest of your life, keep reading. What if you could gain knowledge about how to liberate yourself from that dependency if possible? Thyroid nodules are now more common, as well as cystic acne, ovarian and prostate cancers, heart problems, central nervous system disorders, and, brain tumors. People are being diagnosed with Bipolar, Schizophrenia, and GAD, in numbers never seen before. You have help-you are not "**crazy!**"

**Blood tests and scans are wonderful but they are not everything!**

People are suffering **needlessly; the solution is not difficult. Healing your thyroid gland, is about detoxification and regeneration!** Many will never make the association between thyroid problems and heart issues like Tachycardia that could be remedied and prevented for a great many people. We have far too many thyroid problems and disease codes because **it is not profitable to be *cured*, nor well within, but, it is your birthright.**

Are you suffering with **anxiety, migraines**, and a you want and ***need*** to be alone? Are these feelings affecting your relationships, job/business? **Have you been tested, sometimes extensively and found to have no thyroid problems?** Many people just cannot get to **sleep** and stay sleeping, they often end up using just about anything to get some **sleep**.

**Autoimmune issues** are also reversible, they are often the result of **multi-generational aspects of thyroid imbalance.** I will introduce you to looking at your own multigenerational factors and spot signs of thyroid imbalances in family members.

You will find value with this book because you can detox and heal *without an expensive diet plan and feeling like you are starving yourself. You will learn far more than perhaps what you planned and you will find the truth.*

# CHAPTER ONE - WHY DETOX?

Just about everyone I know can benefit from detoxification. Most people wanted some guidance about how to do it, and, how to feel good again. Unique experiences in my life brought clarity about detoxification, regenerating health, and reversing disease.

Fortunately, I happened to learn about a series of classes in the 1980s taught by Pamela Masters in Los Gatos, California about raw foods and how she had reversed her own cancer. She had trained with The Hippocrates Institute. In the 1980s that was not so common to hear about reversing cancer-she was honest, candid and, humble and the experience for me was life changing.

I began to detoxify, prepare foods and eat the way she had shown us even though it was a big change for me and I had to go out of my way to make it happen. I improved my own health so much that I kept seeking and learning. I found classes at our natural foods store, Bread of Life, in Campbell, California in 1982 where I could learn from the women who were my elders who were making brown rice and cashew or mushroom gravy with steamed vegetables, and using spices and other seasonings I had never heard of back then. Shepard's Pie and other dishes were delicious, simple to make and in class, I was able to watch somebody make one, then I felt much more confident in making one myself.

One cup of real chai from India Joze in Santa Cruz and I quickly replaced coffee and took a food preparation course from them as well! All of this that I was learning and welcoming into my life was upgrading to say the least. I began to feel more connected, intelligent, intuitive and to spend more time in outdoors and moving my body, instead of just being inside or at a store shopping, or any of the ways we live and keep ourselves busy. While out in San Francisco one day at a Greenpeace store in 1987, I asked about what was new and intriguing at the store and I was pointed to new video by John Robbins: Diet for a New America! At this time, his video impressed me so much, it brought tears to my eyes and I was so thankful for it that I bought many copies and I gave them to friends and family, asking them to pass them around and make sure people had the truth about the factory farming of animals, I was horrified about what was happening and what we just considered "food."

Of course, in the beginning you could have called me a young and very impressionable, but I was also in college and I experienced profound positive change with my ability to read, comprehend and have plenty of energy. I began to notice in the 1980s how much people were suffering needlessly after I had applied what I was learning and, I was eager to give back so that everybody could feel this way! All the pounds of pain came off and my skin and hair completely changed over time. I had a more positive outlook on life and much more energy and flexibility. The food and lifestyle changes were without a doubt upgrading me.

Pamela taught us in her series of classes, about detoxification and eating in a way that gave us energy, clarity, kept us healthy, and free from disease. Not only did we learn why we need to detox and from what, but also what the body needs from food to heal. She had reversed cancer in herself and I was absolutely amazed! Initially, I was not all that interested in attending her classes, nor did I really have the money in my budget to do so, but the young man who caught up with me at West Valley College just kept insisting I go, and, I finally made a last minute decision to attend the class as I was told I could come to the first one and then, make my decision about committing to the series - I came to the first class, and, sat there eyes wide open and my jaw, dropped as I listened with Pamela about her journey and what she had learned from Hippocrates at that time. I believe that her course changed my entire life. I too want to give back with all the gathering I have done now for these many decades. When I went to a foraging workshop with Dr. T (Dr. Tel-Oren), last year in Wisconsin, he remarked in a very genuine way that I ran like a 15 year old. My body at age 56 right now is flexible, strong and durable. I am looking forward to sharing with you how you can look and feel this way too and, heal your thyroid.

I have consulted with a wide range of all types of people for years, observed diseases reversed, cured entirely, including thyroid disease, Myasthenia Gravis, cancer, Diabetes, Lupus-many of these were *technically* autoimmune. People experience metabolic/weight changes, integumentary/skin, became radiant and blemish free, Asthma, Allergies, Eczema, Psoriasis, Infertility, PCOS, Endometriosis, Fibroids, Fibromyalgia, Bipolar, ADHD, ODD, all reduced or entirely reversed. Also important, moods improved, no more dandruff, sweating issues, constipation was no longer a reality, and doctor visits ended with a smile, among many other beautiful improvements. Thyroid healing is not difficult-I will show you just how to do it.

When you detoxify your body you allow your body to shed inflammation, toxins and the body can eventually eliminate the lumps, bumps, cysts and nodules. There is no mystery as to why we have so many cysts, they are a **byproduct** of our daily habits. There are habits we keep that most people do not even think about twice. I will cover these for you step-by-step so that you can make the changes you are comfortable with and to the degree that you apply them you will experience healing.

It has been decades now that I have experienced detoxification and keeping myself healthy. I have realized how we create, store, and produce problems with holding onto congested matter in our digestive tract-what even a sluggish elimination can do. I realize that everything I put into my mouth has a direct effect on how I feel and experience life as well as everything I put into my Mind-my thoughts relates to how I feel.

Certain foods will bring down my vibration, or my energy and yet we crave them often because of memories we have and associations we have made with the experiences generated around them. I have taken responsibility for healing myself through several instances, including a major diagnosis which called me to task to not only stand by what I know, but also to use it diligently and prepare a plan that I had to stick with 100% as anyone would have perceived Ovarian Carcinoma as life threatening, and, I had the medical "evidence," in the form of all they're testing and checking and, I had to trust myself and what I believe in-as well as a child to raise, I had to make peace with life on a whole new level and get crystal clear about what I represent and what I do, and in these times when you are faced with more, it will make you, or break you.

Now, if I get off track for a bit with my daily habits-food, water, exercise, and, what I know provides me with self-love and health, I experience a downshift and, kind of suffer for it. You can, like I have, gently get yourself back into the habits of taking care of you-I am here now, encouraging you because I want you to succeed in healing your own thyroid, and to realize how powerful you truly are!

Detoxification does not have to be painful, nor frustrating, it can also be quite enjoyable and liberating. Your body moves the toxins which could be heavy metals, mucoid plaque hanging out in your colon from years of overeating, stored emotions in the tissues of your body-chemicals from body care products, parasites, yeast, and of course, congestion and mucous from many of the foods and drinks that most people consume.

**When we detox, ideally we eat foods that are easier to digest: simple foods, and we reduce overeating more easily with the mineral suggestions I am going to give you as you read further so you can curb that runaway appetite** almost all of us had at one time. You could even occasionally taking a day or two to juice fast. Your body knows what to do, even if you feel intimidated right now—stay with me and I will show you simply and easily. Massage, walking and exercise help the body to get toxins moving on out! Massage therapy is ideal on many levels, including keeping your mood up as you detox and helping to move your lymph and get blood and oxygen flow to your muscles. It is a detox in itself! I obtained massage therapy certification in 1997 in Los Gatos, California where I learned some big insights with Stuart Grace, our instructor for the program, and, we were all blessed to have Alaya Chikley from Upledger who knows a great deal about Cranial Sacral Therapy within our group; she gave us some instruction about *still point* and calming the body and mind as well as her passion: healing from the heart! Our body holds information, stress, and, tension, not just physically, but also energetically.

The body and energy field have much information that is shared with a Practitioner. I began to combine all that I gathered with much of what I learned as a young girl with my grandmother; as well as incorporate what I learned from my mother about how the mind works and how our belief affects our outcome. She used to tell me that if she could see it in the mind, it would likely happen. That was the mid 1960s and I now realize how learning from the elders and the 'old ways' has significantly aspected my life's work which became about helping people to **remember** how we have always healed ourselves.

A few years later while working at a Waldorf School for a year as my son attended, I went to American School of Herbalism and took coursework, some of it taught by licensed acupuncturists and others by world famous Herbalists: Michael Tierra and Christopher Hobbs. Herb walks, sage walks at UCSC, getting in touch with plants with a whole new perspective and helped me to transition from what most plant based eaters were doing which was eating a lot of starch. Around 1996, I became more acquainted with Traditional Chinese Medicine, "TCM," and experienced it for myself for several years. I brought my son for Tuina, when he was a baby, which is another type of subtle massage and over a few years, I experienced and benefited from acupuncture for clearing liver stagnation, spleen issues, and opening energy meridians-it's likely where I picked up some of my ways and terminology.

I began to realize medicine that put together many aspects along with my intuitive sensing. I began helping people reverse disease quite actively. In February of 2003 I opened a shop where I combined massage, energy, consultations and **I freely gave a great many medical intuitive and other insights that were given to me as gifts to my clients** who were paying for a massage. I taught over 20 classes and courses and, I gave free presentations about reversing cancer and healing thyroid. I hold myself to a very high standard and I never mixed medicine with my ever drinking alcohol, nor on any substances of any kind. I also faced a lot of doubt, and skepticism about my deep sensing and medical intuitive gifts, yet I did not stop and I never charged a penny for it.

Part of why I share some of this in the beginning before we get to the heart of Detox & Heal Your Thyroid, is because people are very resistant to change and they can feel much more comfortable to stay where they are and complain versus actually make real life change. There are people who want to live healthy and they truly enjoy life and they are eager to learn.

If you are not actively seeking out knowledge, wanting to expand your dreams, your gifts, and your consciousness than you are just existing. If you are just existing then you are not participating with life and one of the ways you will experience this is with thyroid problems. Thyroid is the gland within your neck and your neck is one of the most vulnerable parts of your body-a connector and communicator with mind and physical existence.

Having a thyroid imbalance symbolically reveals how your mind interprets your life experience.

I will cover detoxification, food, lifestyle, Mind Body, environment, and more so that you have a clear understanding of why we have so many thyroid problems with so many people today. There is not just one reason, one food, one pill, nor one program that will cause your thyroid problem, nor heal it. Your thyroid will regenerate with a concerted effort. Read the book and I will guide you step-by-step as **we make a written plan for you in a journal or a composition book so it is in writing and you can turn to it.**

# CHAPTER TWO - WHY DO WE HAVE THYROID PROBLEMS?

Your thyroid gland is a part of you that is **experiencing input** along your life journey. All the joys, stresses, foods, habits, products, lack of sleep, drugs, medications, smoking, vaping, and, throat clearing. Think of it as the thermostat or, the governor: thyroid keeps your temperature just right, your weight in proportion, it has to do with your moods, emotions and more than people have ever realized, until now! Thy Rod and Thy Staff they comfort me, if they are not well, you are uncomfortable! I think the rod thy rod was our thyroid! The staff was our spine leading to our cranium-our thyroid is near our cervical spine.

We are stressed on many levels-We are not living according to our nature. Physical stress happens from radiation, not having minerals, vitamins, and, enzymes we need-foods that are modified and designed to be addicting-eating has become almost recreational. Because we sit and watch screens and game for far too many hours. We go to work and sit and stress mentally, and, we stress because we long for our freedom. Stress affects us mentally because we are busy, but not really satisfied with life. Emotionally, because of our way of life and the expectations that we all have! We can do something about it, which is why I wrote Detox & Heal Your Thyroid. You can put together a plan with me, step by step, and experience relief.

Would we have thyroid problems today if we were living according to our nature? I do not believe we would. We would be walking more, and not living in homes filled with electromagnetic fields, electro-pollution, living near cell phone towers, (RF), eating synthetic foods and consuming many brominated products. We would have never allowed drinks that are yellow, red, green and orange because somebody made a profit at the cost of our children, parents and elders that are fed toxic products.

Many of our drinks are sold in endocrine disrupting plastic, as well as in aluminum cans. Drinking highly acidic, drinks like coffee every single day will definitely bring you trouble with your thyroid. Many drinks targeted to our young people are the worst offenders. Bromine has been found in certain soft drinks as well as sports recovery drinks that are harmful to your thyroid like Mt. Dew, Fanta Orange, Squirt, and Powerade and Gatorade have a flavor that is made with **brominated vegetable oil** "BVO." One of my favorites as a teenager was Fresca and that too, has BVO. There are certain chemicals that are a direct hazard to your thyroid gland and BVO is one of them. How many people are now placing 12 packs of Mt. Dew and some of these other "drinks" into their grocery carts?

We are using many products that we do not give a second thought about using: hair products, body washes, fragrances, colognes, hair dye, perms, lye, to name a few that contain harmful ingredients and, produce problems for your thyroid. But there's more, products that produce off-gassing like much of our carpets, furniture, beds, RVs and more. What if more people knew that spraying many of our foods with bromine like we often do with many of our berries is directly harmful to our thyroid.

**Think about thyroid imbalance as the body reacting to being choked!** In original medicine we are thankful for the the opportunity of thyroid imbalance to increase our awareness of what we must do. We can stop being choked, as it costs us all to lose nutrients like important minerals that used to be in our food, and soils. We can observe our way of life and how it may feel as though we are choked down with contaminants in our air, clothing, and around us in many ways. Thyroid issues are epidemic and pandemic at this time, because of our need to be able to speak our truth, be heard and feel like our voice matters. **Being stressed produces thyroid imbalance.**

When our food becomes less nutrient dense with enzymes, minerals and vitamins, we no longer fund the body with what it needs. **Our thyroid and entire body needs iodine.** Much of our **thyroid hormones are built with iodine**, and T3 and T4 are made with three and four parts iodine respectively. I am looking forward to our journey when later in the book I cover more about iodine and how to use it.

Most of us lack bioavailable iodine, and, likely because of the convenience of grab and go. With anxiety the result of thyroid problems, we are easily overwhelmed, and have trouble with attention and organization. Why I help people with ADHD which also has a thyroid root cause. It feels like too much to prepare real food and even those who do are confused with what it takes to stay healthy. Anxiety and depression does us in and causes more impulsive behaviors which make it easy to keep violating our thyroid gland by grabbing a pizza out a drive up window, or to take home and bake, or a quick sandwich on the hot shelf at the local corner store. The quick burrito is faster, easier and often less expensive on the budget so we rationalize that it is healthy and we saved time, money and cleaning the kitchen. We eat behind the wheel. We want more convenient foods and people now request fruits without seeds. Most of my older clients in their 70s and a few that are 80 are in great shape because they still prepare food at home and they lived during a time when food was not as toxic as it is today. Keep good habits: start with small ones, like waking up and just being thankful for life, drink some water and carry your food with you. You will need to obtain a couple small dollar store composition books or a journal, so write down that you need to get those or gather some paper so you can begin to make this awesome plan with me to help you!

It is important that I bring this up as well: many people have developed unnatural fears. Fear of the ticks outside so they do not get out and walk on a trail in nature. Fears of being in the sun with sun cancer scares causes them to apply sunscreen to "protect" themselves. People fear their high blood pressure and take blood pressure medications, or who have depression or SAD and take "Vitamin D." Yet we do much of our healing by walking, being out in Nature, and we feed from the sun, in moderation. Sunscreen is toxic, I have never applied it and I won't and you deny your skin healing from the sun. People are concerned about skin cancer for good reason: the fear generated which sells products and creates reliance on checking and, finding. While skin cancer is real, it is often the result of a body that cannot eliminate through the skin and, a person who needs to detoxify.

Our modern way of life has caused the inability to detoxify from our skin and, we are now afraid of the sun. We are clogged and congested with mucous. We do not walk and allow them to release through the skin. We keep covering up the symptoms that are doing their best to inform: underarm stink, bowel movements stink, urine is bubbly and smells, the skin erupts and tries to discharge toxins and we treat that with acne medications and call it 'normal' for teens to experience acne in the same way we call it normal for women to have hot flashes as they go through the changes in life. For many decades now we have progressively caused our own demise. We demand faster, more convenient and spend more time facing a blue screen and then, eat ice cream. I know you will value a great part of this book and your plan with me step by step is to become more present, real and authentic. More comfortable and well.

When you are outside and, near the sea you **get doses of iodine mist from the ocean saltwater.** If people begin to consume more prepackaged and convenience foods, they miss out because they do not contain the sunlight which has been photosynthesized and is contained in seaweeds, fresh green plants, raw nuts and seeds, certain flowers and what we call herbs and spices. We do best when we enjoy tea, a variety of salads, real and organic sun ripened foods. These foods give us energy, minerals and they help aid our thyroid gland with more bioavailable minerals and trace nutrients that are not found in processed foods. For most people, real sun-ripened foods are not a part of their daily diets like they once were. Young adults often live entirely on sandwiches, frozen foods, and grab and go foods from the deli and convenience stores. Even recently when sharing meals with people I suggest that we get outside and sit down and eat together. Begin to notice your daily habits.

I prepare a blended drink that is easier to digest after fasting all night and if I am able I hold off until later morning it allows for a bit of a longer fast from the night before to reduce my caloric intake just a bit. This also gives you more energy than quickly eating and filling up because we feel we have to have breakfast; we don't if we do not feel inclined to eat first thing in the morning. I think you may like this like I do, and take it along with you in a recycled jar or other container.

**Blended Drink - A Morning Favorite!**

1 Cantaloupe cut into chunks with skin removed blended with 1/4 cup filtered water
2 frozen organic bananas
1 Tablespoon of Gelatinized MACA root

You will know you have thyroid problems if you are cold often, or if you are overheating. Tired all the time and you have lethargy, unusual or no sex drive or libido, and there are hundreds of ways most people know and once you become familiar you can spot them a mile away. Nearly all of them respond to the same cure: Detox & Heal. Remember, to cure, is to relieve your symptoms and feel well, it does not state in the dictionary that you remove the diagnosis code, it says that you relieve yourself of the symptoms. People stand in awe all the time about people being cured, why is this? Because we do not become well unless we are willing to detox and heal.

Some of the factors related to having thyroid problems are nuclear radiation leaks, toxic spills, lead, toxic heavy metals, they are affecting our entire genetic makeup, our bones, muscles, cells, tissues, organs and glands. Children and younger people are experiencing and being diagnosed with thyroid problems. We can begin to observe on a multigenerational level so that we can learn from our families, and, we can learn from history and mistakes that have been made. We can also prevent, and prepare our younger family members.

**As many as perhaps 90% of the people in the area where I live now in what is often called a "Goiter Belt," are experiencing a thyroid imbalance of some sort-most of which are not officially diagnosed.** Underlying the Parkinson's Disease, the Kidney Disease, Fibromyalgia, Lupus, ADHD and in my opinion, ODD, and many more a diagnosis is an undetected thyroid imbalance and a need to detox and heal.

Thyroid problems manifest in many ways, with a variety of symptoms.Our medical system is specialized and compartmentalized today. Someone may be diagnosed with a gynecological, digestive, integumentary (skin), structural or in other ways which may have a thyroid root cause, particularly, PCOS, Endometriosis, Infertility and miscarriages.

It seems obvious to me now that if we continue to treat, medicate, surgically remove and kill off with RAI, the offending problem, the source or the root of the problem is never addressed and later, we often have a new and different diagnosis which is compounded and more difficult to unwind and reverse, unless you are consulting with somebody with a great deal of experience.

# CHAPTER THREE - MULTIGENERATIONAL ASPECTS OF THYROID IMBALANCE

Thyroid problems were a part of my life and, they are affecting some of my closest family members. Two men in my family have been diagnosed with thyroid cancer. One family member has committed suicide years after a diagnosis and surviving it by many years. I became very familiar with the mental and emotional aspects of thyroid disease.

Thyroid imbalances can produce anxiety, insomnia, depression and without detoxification can lead to what could be diagnosed as Bipolar, Schizophrenia and be the root cause preceding suicide.

I can see clearly where thyroid imbalance struck many members of my family in different ways. In a page of your composition book or journal, create a section for multigenerational considerations and then, write down maternal on one side and paternal on the other and the names of your grandparents on each side, then your parents on each side and underneath each, write down what they experienced, whether obesity, goiter, thyroid, cancer, and what type, diabetes and anything else.

Take a look at pictures of yourself, your family, and other relatives; whatever you have or can look up online but observe in a different way now, specifically, look at the eyes of the people in the pictures for tightness, bulging, eyelid puffiness, swollen faces, body size, whether pencil thin, average, or obese.

Ask about relatives and dig into your family history check for goiters, dwarfism, giantism, scoliosis, left handers, breech births, people in your family with high or low blood pressure, high or low intelligence, mental retardation, tooth problems, overbite, diseases at the time of death that were noted, and note what you find about multigenerational history in your own family.

Teenagers and young adults with a multigenerational history and mothers who were thyroid and mineral deficient are now commonly showing up with thyroid imbalance emotionally and mentally at a younger ages. The children today have more Autism, ADHD, ODD, and learning disabilities. What do we do? We need to get people doing the detox & healing themselves instead of medicating.

There are other factors to our Multigenerational thyroid problems that involved parental exposure to radiation due to nuclear atomic testing which took place for decades in Nevada alone, but also other places, and nuclear leakages today like Fukushima and Chernobyl. There are multigenerational issues produced by lineages with lack of iodine and minerals and exposures.

When people live near toxic industrial factories, paper mills and gross polluters, and they have a poor diet, a high starch diet, consume wheat and dairy, drink soft drinks and lots of coffee, do not walk, and come from multigenerational thyroid deficits and lack of iodine the result was commonly: Crohn's Disease, severe colon issues, and Paranoid Schizophrenia but there are a great many more diagnosis codes they are being invented every single day.

Up North, in Minnesota, there are much higher incidences of mental health, suicide, cancer, neurological syndromes and disease. Despite doing my best to educate people in these small pockets of the state, people would continue to spend hundreds of dollars on bottles. People need to be willing to change their way of life, they must be open minded enough to hear it, live it and do it. If not, it's a waste of breath and energy.

### Lipoma & Buffalo Humps

**If you are experiencing a Lipoma there is a need to detox and heal. And, there is a need for minerals, especially Iodine.** Iodine will cause your body to start discharging the cysts, lumps, bumps, fatty cysts and benign tumors in your organs, but, I caution you to read through the book and get your journal or composition book so that you note each step of the way and you write down your personal goals as I want you to be more successful as soon as possible and not be dissatisfied. Instead of reaching for iodine right this minute, please, get some paper and start writing down the aspect of detoxification that you can and will do step by step so that you body can eliminate the toxic material more successfully.

Lipomas can appear on the body, neck, torso, and other places and they can appear on any animal. You are an animal, a mammal specifically.

Lipoma and Buffalo Humps found behind the thyroid gland on the neck are a collection of adipose tissue, a clump of cells that cannot detoxify on their own. It is a signal to me that you are not walking, moving enough stagnation by walking and eliminating properly now or at some time in your life. And, you are not sweating enough. You may be sweating now, but at some time you were not. It can indicate that you are or have been eating wheat, dairy, factory farmed meats or that you are exposed to some environmental toxins. The largest tool for you right now is walking every single day, for an hour or longer, even if you divide that up into several walks.

If you are able, observe in your own family and ask questions. Lipoma behind the neck is commonly associated with thyroid gland imbalances. I am now seeing this on younger and younger people. While doing massage I found this on girls in high school and I see this on younger and younger people which is not a good sign. With detoxification your body will cease holding onto the lipoma.

You will have to do internal as well as external detoxification with lipomas. We have to remove stress to the degree possible, detoxify the body and the mind and begin to put in food as medicine. Often, removing the wheat and dairy alongside detoxification and then adding in missing minerals will produce what many would call miracles! Most people are missing magnesium and sulfur in their diets. To cause your own body to detoxify to remove the lipoma you must do some massage, eat foods high in sulfur, use some DMSO topically with aloe vera and you can also prepare sulfur and Epsom salt treatments, which I cover in consultations individually so that I do not make the book too detailed about Lipomas and Buffalo Humps. They are a part of thyroid imbalances and specifically mineral deficit: iodine. Iodine will not work exclusively by itself, so please keep reading and then have your plan written down so that you do it well and do not waste your time and money jumping in too fast. Once you read through detoxification and about the minerals and supplements you will see what I mean.

### Anxiety as an Aspect of Thyroid Imbalance

How many generations of your family experienced anxiety? Whether social anxiety, GAD, Bipolar, or absolutely crippling anxiety that is referred to as Agoraphobia? How many others in your family did not get out around people and enjoy life? Or, were diagnosed with anxiety related disorders? How many were diagnosed with Bipolar or Schizophrenia or other mental health diagnosis? Be sure and make any notes about this in your journal or book.

Have you noticed how much more difficult it is for us to get along with each other? The more anxiety, depression, and stress we have, the less agreeable we are with one another and we begin to do more dividing sadly. Detoxification and healing of your thyroid brings people back together again, so that they can possibly be calmer, more loving and present. Perhaps that can happen through you reading this book and helping another family member and preventing the children from following the same path as their parent or parents with drug abuse, anxiety, and mental health issues that can be observed and a plan put together for them now as prevention planning.

If you have a child or teen at home now with horrid oppositional defiant behaviors "ODD," if they are willing you can begin with an HTMA and test their hair which is available on my website: **www.naturallywithkaren.com** and then put together a plan for their detox at least from the 3 foods and also get minerals into them. They can sleep better and focus better and it will be a positive change for all!

How many people reading this right now have family that cannot spend time together? We  cannot get along. Families barely limping along with tons of stress due to other family members with an OCD diagnosis, or struggle with perfectionism? All of these branches are from the same tree! The Root of all of these are a need to detoxify, add minerals and thyroid imbalance. But most people would not know that would they? And, wouldn't it be nice if we could rid ourselves of these problems? We can! **But, you have to actually do the work**, *or, hire somebody to consult with to do some of the hand holding and guiding for you.* It may take up to 2 weeks to see dramatic differences in inattentiveness, compulsiveness, fear, anxiety, depression, and foul moods that can take over-if you do not make a plan it will get worse!

Would most people make the connection with a parent with thyroid cancer and a child with Generalized Anxiety Disorder or ADHD? I know the answer because I not only experienced this in my close family, but, I see it all the time with my clients. I encourage you to open your mind to this and I realize it takes some getting used to, it did not happen overnight for me. I wrote this book to **distill** a lot of my learning and experience consulting with people so that you have it for yourself and loved ones and don't spend years like I did to figure it out.

When Mom has anxiety or OCD, and the child has ADHD it becomes even more difficult to sit down and figure things out when you are faced with stress, behaviors and complaints from teachers right now and you need a solution immediately. Medication is what most people know! And, they only know that route singularly. This is very confusing to parents who really want to avoid the antidepressant or anti anxiety medication route. I will assure you that most of the time, when young people are detoxed, the gut healed, and off a few of the foods, and onto a few minerals, and you get them outside walking (no small feat in today's world), they improve dramatically they are like an entirely different personality.

Getting out and walking is an absolute must to detox & heal!

Over the years, I have often taken people out with me and the dogs, (The Pack), and we walk in nature, which is a good mental release. I realize that if people have a week or a month to experience this way of life, then they could do it themselves on their own. I affectionately joke about a Pack It Up Camp. Walking, a little bit of real yoga, simple and real food, sunshine, outdoors, away from screens, being real-amazing how this restores people.

## Getting Started

What you will achieve by reading and preparing a plan is that your throat and thyroid will detoxify and heal and your mind will become calmer. You will heal your gut, and begin to digest and eliminate much more efficiently and with less pain. You can sit down and listen in conversation or while reading a book because once you replace missing minerals and iodine you can be more fully present, authentic and in the present moment with people. Instead of nearly everyone around you looking like the deer in the headlights, and with rapid speech, they will begin to settle down and be here, now.

**You do not have to live the rest of your life with mental and emotional difficulties that are often interpreted as strictly mental health issues,** with Detox & Heal Your Thyroid if you choose to put my suggestions into practice in your life you will see profound results! Much of what you suffer from now, will no longer plague you: the weight will fall off, you will sleep again, your anxiety will reduce then disappear, **your thyroid nodules will shrink**, and your body will heal. This is how and why I got started. As a Mother I was motivated because of the love I have for my child. I needed to make things better for him! He did not deserve an exhausted, screaming, angry Mom a part of his childhood. We can become somebody we never dreamed we could ever become.

Without a diagnosis should you get started with a detox so you can heal your own body, mind and spirit? Yes, you should! Other issues like hair loss, hair thinning, early male pattern baldness, dyslexia, ODD, ADHD, weird skin rashes, dandruff, skin tags, dry skin, hair and nails, ridges on your nail beds, experiencing more colds and flu, allergies, Asthma, weight gain or a lot of weight loss, feeling as though you may have parasites which is very common, having alcohol or drug abuse problems. Needing to smoke cannabis daily and vape or consume cannabis to get through the day with anxiety or depression, seasonal affective disorder "SAD." These are just a few but there are a lot more! Detox & Heal Your Thyroid will definitely help you with any of these.

Did you know that thyroid issues are commonly linked with heart problems? Same with Chronic Fatigue Syndrome, Irritable Bowel Syndrome, and, Sleep Apnea.

Many of us have **autoimmune issues** related to our thyroid gland like Hashimoto's Disease but before we had an official diagnosis we had been given warnings, and now, our own immune system is attacking itself. Your immune system is your cells, tissues and organs that defend you from attack. War language is used for conditions of our mind and body, we speak of attacking, battling, defending, conquering and killing our lack of ease?

**Autoimmune is not forever!** Nearly everyone I speak with knows somebody they care about who has an autoimmune disease. If your immune system is not functioning as it is supposed to, **it has degenerated**-it's that simple. it is confused.

**Where do we start?** Start with the Pre-Detox and keep reading, then, get the journal or the composition book and let's write down your plan as we go along.

Whether you have long term autoimmune issues, or a simple thyroid problem, I wrote this book so most everyone has a recipe or plan and can achieve stellar results yourself. I wanted to make it affordable for everybody to find ways to bring balance back into their lives. Getting the book out gives a lot of information and costs less than individual personalized consultations with me. The book will take you through what most everyone will need to successfully detox and heal your thyroid. Sometimes we need coaching or consultations to help us on a **personal** level-you do what works best for you! However you are best supported. I am here for you.

Autoimmune issues are not impossible to heal, but due to the length of time they have become habituated within they are a bit more resistant to leave their defense post! It is possible but there are Mind Body aspects as well which must be heard and redirected.

**Think of this as Graduation!**

Denatured, devitalized, and genetically modified foods are increasingly being consumed by people of all ages. Our WIC and other food programs that are distributed by agencies to assist mothers and children in the school food programs are further complicating our lives as they are heavy with traditional nutrition slated with approved lists with items like **whole grains and dairy**, while they are low in content on any real fresh fruit and vegetables. Many Dietitians and Diet Counselors have not changed their programs despite ample evidence that **wheat and gluten dramatically elevate glycemic index and congest and harm the body**, particularly the throat, thyroid and the gut. Becoming aware is Graduating into healthful and, sustainable diets for personal and environmental wellness. After many years, I realize most people want to do this but they have never seen what getting off these foods would look like. This is why I suggest that you get your weekly groceries or go twice per week to the store and get fresh produce and bring it home and use it! That blended drink in the morning, taking your own lunch if possible or go home and make it. You can always make a salad, steamed vegetables, chickpea patties and fresh avocado or guacamole, spiral sliced veggies and a great sauce or a fresh pot of easy to make soup and utilize some of your seaweeds we will cover a bit further on! You can do it! Always have a snack or two in your purse, or your car and then you are less inclined to pull over and grab the convenience store foods or eat what is placed in front of you at a business or school meeting or book club. It would be great if we did not have to graduate from these food chemicals, that trigger our brain and cause us so many problems, but we must!

With detoxing and healing you will experience considerable improvement of your thyroid, **less throat clearing, mucous that people spit up all the time, and, in the shower,** and all the way around a better quality of life! Once you see it with your own eyes you will be entirely amazed as I have time after time! Radiance, beautiful skin, higher intelligence and function and deep healing. Most people do not even realize how often they clear their throat and they often attribute throat clearing to something else other than congestion and thyroid issues.

**Love, is consideration and, it is grounding!** Green plant-based foods are love! Those grown in mineral rich soil are very grounding for us. Fruits are exciting and for this reason we eat them earlier in the day and vegetables are grounding and they calm us later in the day.

Walking in Nature is grounding: to be out amongst the respiration of the trees, plants and the beauty of Nature, the added plus is that we receive negative ions from being close to moving water, and we move peristalsis by pressing down as we walk on the bottoms of our feet moving our digestion and stimulating our organs internally. Sunlight, walking and Nature as well as being near large lakes and the ocean are recharging and, this is why you like to be at the beach or by the lake or river to relax. You are feeding yourself, and your cells, naturally.

People with hypothyroidism which is the most common are mineral and iodine deficient. Their thermostat is not functioning well.

# CHAPTER FOUR - STRESS & THYROID

Stress and thyroid imbalance do not mix! Stress greatly harms your thyroid. Mothers are a special consideration as I have learned as we must supply baby with minerals and we are without enough ourselves it can affect us greatly in a negative way. We become very depleted and exhausted to the point of becoming someone we do not recognize.

How do we go from devoted mother to raging, angry and unpredictable? While babies were in utero, moms give up pounds of their own mineral supply to their developing baby and if they are in short supply themselves they will feel the pull from their own body: bones, and especially their gums and teeth.

I learned from direct experience and I always hope I can reach a woman who is planning a pregnancy in pre-conception or a pregnant mother so we can prevent and protect her.

Summer brings warm or hot weather and unplanned detoxification when mucous begins to thin and drain from the body. People complain about the winter because they have an intolerance to the cold. It is easy to see now why some people relate that they just love the cold and walk around in a t shirt all winter because their body is racing and overheated much of the time you can see the red ruddy facial skin and how they flush when they get anywhere warm.

Overeating causes great wear and tear to your gut and your body-especially elimination. It is epidemic. We keep eating as our brain tries to obtain more minerals and energy and, because of the way the wheat is designed and many of the food chemicals that cause you to eat even when you are not hungry. First step is to become aware and mindful of overeating. Also be aware and note down in your plan if you heard the message to "clean your plate," while growing up and how this may have affected you?

## Thyroid Gland & Our Mouth

Thyroid issues, stress and dental work go hand in hand! More issues to note in your plan here: If you have toxic heavy metals in your mouth, with fillings, crowns, root canals, and other dental work. This is another opportunity by taking inventory of your mouth. Take a look inside and see if you have any of the silver mercury amalgam fillings. If you do, be aware that they have interfered with your thyroid gland. Please write that down on your plan to heal your thyroid. I had a mouthful and had mine removed in 2004-2005. No easy task, but it is doable, I had 23 fillings at the age of 12 and I felt certain that they were causing anxiety. At that time, I could not afford a biologic dentist and I went with a local dentist that I felt did a great job. I stayed present and thankful for getting them out of my mouth without a huge amount of pain! Many people also got large deep expansive fillings as that was the way things were done years ago. There is mercury, copper and other materials in the amalgam fillings that are harmful to you, and your thyroid gland. You can also ask the dentist which tooth number is filled or has dental work done to it and look up the meridian of each tooth based on the tooth number online. Each tooth has a corresponding organ meridian for the body.

When you have a sluggish thyroid you can experience a thicker, fatter tongue which will evidence a thyroid imbalance. During consults with clients I asked people if they ever felt as though their tongue was too big for their mouth. I am often surprised by the numbers of people who say that they do feel this way. Always check your tongue as it will give you good information about you and your internal health. The scalloped tongue is usually thick and fat and it begins to become crowded amongst the teeth.

Another thing to do, is take a few moments and look at pictures of yourself as a baby-look to see if you see any puffy or swollen eyelids or facial tissues. Take a look at your children's pictures also to see if you see swelling and puffy eyelids. Make notes in your book and plan that you have looked over your and family pictures for edema.

If mom is thyroid and mineral deficient, baby or young children can end up Myxedemic. This can also happen with elders as well. It can be brought on by medications and in many ways. Myxedema is a severe hypothyroidism, the heart, blood pressure, body temperature and all are low. This can happen for people who have had their thyroid removed as well.

It is common knowledge today that over 50% of people are not diagnosed as having a thyroid imbalance with venous blood testing. The only problem is that people who do not know will not begin to heal themselves nor prevent other issues from occurring the result of not knowing they have thyroid issues.

Now that you know various signs and symptoms to look for, and are beginning to set up a plan which may include removal of mercury amalgam fillings, and ways to check yourself. If your tongue is thick, fat, and causes you to talk a bit funny, when you visit a doctor, it is called Macroglossia.

I have met with many clients who were certain that their doctors had already checked them for thyroid issues, still, I had noticed their thinning eyebrows, puffy eyelids and heard how they were tired all the time, saw shiners under their eyes, experienced how cold their hands and feet were and how much they dreaded winters coming. I asked them to step over to the mirror at my shop and we took a look at their tongue together and I found that most were already presenting with several hypothyroidism symptoms. Many women who came for consults had a tongue that was swollen and with scalloped edges. If people have a fast thyroid their tongue may be cracked, fissured, red, and the person may tell you their tongue is actually hot, and when the tip of the tongue is very red it indicates a lot of heart heat or that there is a potential problem. White coating indicates digestive issues.

It is common with thyroid issues to produce more caries or cavities and possibly malocclusions of the jaw, which is an overbite where the top teeth or jaw extend over the lower jaw or teeth. This was present in a close family member as well. When it comes to detoxing and healing our thyroid we want to think about not only the products we use everyday to brush and care for our teeth but also the water we use to brush and rinse. In almost every home I visit, children are using toothpaste that contains fluoride and many still receive fluoride treatments at the dentist to "protect," their teeth. It is widely known that fluoride is a neurotoxin. I will be keeping fluoride out of my mouth and I suggest you do the same; especially for children. Since this book is about detoxification, perhaps, keep a gallon of filtered or distilled water in their bathroom just for rising their mouth with a small reusable cup to avoid the chlorine and fluoride of the city water when brushing their teeth. Make a note of this on your plan for yourself to heal your thyroid.

If you are of a certain age you may remember that schools used to distribute fluoride to students in elementary school. I have spoken with many people who have a memory of this happening in their schools when they were young. When I was in school, I remember a tray of small plastic cups with a pink liquid and we were told to take our fluoride treatment.

At one time, fluoride was used as a drug to treat Hyperthyroidism. Fluoride is antagonistic to your thyroid hormone and can mimic the action of Thyrotropin "TSH."For this reason alone I find it inconceivable to use fluoride, particularly with the thyroid issues most of us are suffering from today. It seems to obvious to me, that when somebody has a fast or hyperthyroid there is an urgent need once they have come into the hospital or clinic to stop the fast thyroid and so using radioactive iodine or fluoride make sense to me now as they are halides and they are toxic to the thyroid.

Fluoride is a halide, it can interfere with the function of the thyroid gland. I always recommend seeking a fluoride-free toothpaste, rinses, mouthwashes or any other items for your mouth.

Detox yourself from fluoride by purchasing tooth care products free of fluoride, or making your own tooth products with coconut oil, activated charcoal, baking soda and there are many other ways to clean your teeth and take care of them that are free of halogens. You will find a deeper satisfaction in making your own products as you will know what is inside of them and you are your own quality control!

## The Smoking Chimney

Detox yourself from smoking, whatever it is, cannabis, cigarettes, pipes or other drugs; it causes problems with your throat. Smoking is unnatural and causes your throat and thyroid gland to deal with hot smoke. It is far better if you are healing your thyroid to detoxify yourself from smoking and if you are a cannabis user to consume cannabis in edibles rather than smoke it. I realize many people are very attached to smoking but this is one way to also help heal your thyroid is to consider switching to smoking less or ceasing smoking. While the argument can be made that cannabis is an apoptotic and it is healing, you can also juice it and take it in the form of non-animal butters made into edibles just like with white willow bark it can be taken in capsule form instead of smoking as many people have done.

## The Infant PKU

Did you know that metabolic testing which screens for hypothyroidism is done at the hospitals when a baby is born? One of the ways we are all checked when we are born is through infant testing. If you birthed in a hospital **each baby in the hospital is given the PKU heel stick to check for metabolic issues including hypothyroidism.** Once we are home and as our babies and toddlers develop **we need to look for more obvious and early signs of thyroid or metabolic issues, such as facial swelling, eyelid puffiness, water retention/edema, and delayed ankle reflexes. We can begin to help mothers to avoid the pitfalls of post PARTUM and baby to avoid the developmental issues that could present in childhood but are often dismissed today.** I would love to see wellness exams with mother and baby include education and guidance about minerals, real food and educating families about taking our babies off corn, wheat and dairy as well as most commercial infant formula.

This testing began in 1963 in Massachusetts for metabolic disorders. Phenylketonuria is the basis for the testing and I encourage you to read about this and the testing more fully and learn. Perhaps if mothers had the minerals and clean food, as well as absence of radiation exposure we would no longer need most of these tests. Often, we are told that all these tests are done out of necessity because of genetic mutations.

# CHAPTER FIVE - GUT HEALTH & YOUR THYROID

You want to upgrade your gut so that you can heal yourself and you are able to utilize the nutrients more fully through your digestion. Many of our supplements are capsules and tablets they will not do us much good if our digestive fire is not strong. I see this all the time at the natural foods store with people buying lots of bottles of something they heard about from a friend or on TV.

To the average person who hears the gurgles of the stomach as it is healing and resetting they interpret this as a need to eat more. However, eating first thing in the morning is not the best idea. Your digestion is far stronger later in the day, especially after doing some walking. Yet that break-fast programming is a big part of people's reality. Reducing your calories and waiting to eat a bit later in the day if that works for you is ideal. Beginning your day with freshly prepared juice introduces fresh live enzymes and, fills you up ideally full of energy! Raw fruit, and a warm chai if it is winter and cold outside. In order to strengthen your gut you can also curb eating within hours of going to sleep so that your sleep time not interrupted by digesting and the need to eliminate. Be sure to write down in your plan that you want to really get your digestive fire up by reducing consumption of food if you are eating is excessive.

Eliminating wheat from your diet redirects your attention to other sources of food that are not made of wheat, or gluten found in rye and barley. A regular diet of wheat, rye and barley contribute to a weakened gut, digestive and elimination systems as well as leaky gut from the way that wheat is now designed. You can read more about wheat in our food section of this book.

Another benefit of healing your belly with detoxification steps and avoiding certain foods, and, lifestyle changes is having the ability to know when you are truly hungry, vs. recreational eating. Not constantly eating because your mind is seeking comfort. As we get into the detoxification and food, you will see why preparation and advance planning along with the need to carry food with you will help you to strengthen your gut and stay strong! This means that you gear up to learn the art of food preparation.

Even on the road, you can prepare foods which means that they do not have to be cooked over heat. Examples are spiral sliced squash, beets, onions, and lots of the cheesecakes and pies I make are entirely raw and do not need to be heated. Raw foods will give you more enzymes and vitamins most of the time over cooked foods, they are simple and quick and you almost never need a recipe. A **food rhythm** is important to healing your gut because you are eating what is local and seasonal to the extent possible, and use what you have and you use it to prepare something simple. I have some pictures of my food rhythm on my website. You begin to engage with the ease and simplicity of a natural food rhythm. For example, today I had 5 green apples and 4 cucumbers and I juiced them and ate the other 2 cucumbers with a dash of grape seed oil and some sulfur rich black salt and a bit of garlic salt.

Another example, is while I was at a friends house this past weekend, I made a dish to share out of it and a few other things I found to put together on the spot. I had been given one peach, I spotted one zucchini on the table from a garden, and I saw an apple. I washed and cut up the raw fruits and the large squash into small bites and then poured a small amount of some of her real maple syrup over it. I divided it up into 5 small cereal bowls and handed it out so we all ate together. It was delicious and it fed all 5 of us for a late morning meal.

Later that morning there was a pot of local fresh cooked corn that we were going to toss out from the day before and I took it and rinsed it really well, used a cleaver style knife and cut the corn off the cobb and mixed in some soaked raisins, an onion, lemon peel, salt, apple cider vinegar, cayenne and while I don't usually buy or support eating corn, I was able to make a large delicious bowl of food for everyone that was willing to eat the corn- that I usually avoid. All of the wheat items that were brought and on the table where we sat lay untouched.

You will restore gut strength if you do the upcoming pre-detox and quit wheat sooner than later, and you will begin to rapidly lose belly fat, your thyroid will begin to heal as well; but, it will never happen, nor will healing your thyroid gland if you continue to *use* wheat, gluten, nor a heavy grain based diet. Wheat is everywhere, and, it is an addiction. I get it, it means entire *"conversion,"* yet, having an exponentially better life. Letting go of wheat and gluten should be a lifetime decision. The sooner you give it up, the sooner you will see results!

Best to get your peristalsis moving. I cannot emphasize how important this is! Your digestive system is stimulated as you walk through reflex points on your feet. Barefoot walking or flexible, shoes that bend are ideal. Walking in Nature provides a refreshing uplift to the day, as well as long term benefits to moving the blood and the lymph. For all the people who ask me questions about hair fall on quora.com this is one of your best tools. Release mental tension and stress, and move energy and stagnation.

I am thankful when I walk outside with nature, for the beauty of the trees, birds and fresh air. I love the peace and quiet, sounds of nature, and away from environments which are heavy with EMFs (refrigerators, microwaves, heaters, and all our electrical devices plugged in at home or our offices). When you walk and your foot can flex and bend whether barefoot or in flexible shoes, you are moving old digested matter in your colon. In order to have the best possible results from this book, make sure that you walk each day. How long should you walk? That's entirely up to you. When I have my way, I want to be outside for hours. I know that we all have to start somewhere and you may go out for shorter walks more often, say 3-15 minute walks per day to start? If you cannot get out and walk, then take your shoes off in the warmer weather and sit in a chair outside with your feet on the Earth and get some time where you can touch the Earth. Walking and Earthing barefoot on the Earth will greatly calm you and help you to heal your gut much more quickly.

### Unplugged

Nature time is crucial to your healing! As you take this journey with me, you too will cherish time spent outdoors versus inside away from sunlight, fresh air, and noticing the sounds of the birds. You will begin to gain a calm and present mind by making this a daily habit. Once you set a goal of walking a mile a day you will feel so good. It's a mental release. Now, increase the time you spend walking in Nature gradually, and, **be 'unplugged.'** **While it is super productive on one level to listen to an audible book or course, and multitask, you miss out on the presence and beauty of nature if you do too much at one time.** Having more time unplugged makes you become more aware of a culture that is driving you to become a virtual consumer, game player and busy all the time. **Just be**, move your body, clear congestion and stagnant energy, listen to the birds and notice the trees. The more time we spend indoors will cause you to become more prone to stay inside isolating which is so common with thyroid disease. Clients and close family have become recluse and begin to pull away from people and events, go outside or make plans with people. It is very common when you do not feel well physically nor emotionally to connect with people except through a computer screen. This is something we can improve and reverse.

**Here is what I recommend to get the most from this book and**

**heal your own thyroid:**

Read through the book first. Next, get yourself a **composition book** from the store, even the dollar store-write down a few ways you feel comfortable to start. Perhaps even get yourself a second composition book and make that your **Food Diary** so you can transition out of some of the foods on the detox and food section of the book. This way you will remember what you need to do by turning to your composition book and food diary each day, you won't get overwhelmed nor frustrated by forgetting as we all do from time to time, especially with thyroid imbalances. You will have your plan right in front of you and you can make a shopping list from it as well. Note any clay, DE, skin brush, probiotic, foods, filtered water, and supplements you plan to keep on your list so that you are successful and reach your goals!

I speak with a lot of people and I realize that transitioning from some of the foods leave people wondering what they are going to eat, so be sure to sign up for the email list at www.onegreenplanet.org so that recipes come to you! Instead of feeling like you are being converted to a diet plan, see this is clarifying what you eat so that you can detox and cause your thyroid gland to regenerate.

You will experience big improvements upon each step of the journey until we get to your goal!

Texting and Snapchat are awesome technology for lots of reasons. I love receiving a text to request scheduling an appointment, or getting a quick snap from my children, however, to use it exclusively is avoidance. **That avoidance is the isolation that creeps in with thyroid imbalances.**

Not spending time with people in person, or having a telephone call and using a text instead of a phone call is not just a trend with younger folks, it is in part thyroid anxiety. Entire applications are designed catering to our people so that most of their communication is brief.

Many of our young people have anxiety, depression, low energy, fatigue and many have no idea that they have thyroid issues. If you know you have a thyroid imbalance you can relate to much of what I am speaking about and if you have not heard a lot of this before, it begins to sound like I blame everything in the world on your thyroid! I realize it can sound this way, and the reason I made this book centered around detoxification and healing is because I realize the food and lifestyle components. For example, what part of having thinning hair and a poor functioning gut are thyroid and what part are wheat? It could be that 80% of it is wheat and you will know after you cut wheat out and do some detoxing. I just wanted to acknowledge that I do not blame all the problems of the world on your thyroid!

**Detoxification can apply to many aspects of your life.** For one, you can detoxify from watching as much of the news on TV; you can cut back on listening or music videos of the more commercial trap music which is full of negative images or words. I really cherish having a quiet environment most of the time. I do not own a TV since 1985 and I prefer it that way.

Detoxification is also spiritual-allowing yourself to just be at peace: not busy all the time so that your spirit is not so heavy with hearing all the negativity in the world constantly. You can take a social media detox and not scroll through your newsfeed or watch all the current snaps, you can sit down and read a book, like this one and have somebody bring knowledge that will greatly increase your life force energy.

You want to give your body and your thyroid every opportunity to provide you with energy, and a great home for your spirit to reside, it cannot function with stress, toxic foods, toxic water and exposure to unnecessary chemicals in your mouth, your toothpaste, your drinking water if it has chlorine and fluoride in it—then we do better. Not just for us as individuals, which certainly we do first, but for the whole of us. There is no shortage of violence, greed and selfishness in the world but I believe we can reduce some of this by also becoming more healthful and sustainable.

Living your life in the present moment is a gift you can give yourself and others around you. Part of detoxification and healing is to bring comfort and peace into your life and to reduce listening with, participating in, and watching negativity. We do not need to know all the negative events happening in the world and bring our spirits down, which is different from not caring.

Be unplugged for a bit and begin to notice around you quietly and from a place of love observe in a city from a park bench or outside a grocery store and watch the people ambling about in large painful bodies: swollen, obese, with many skin issues, and often speaking about their ailments. All of these people would feel remarkably better if they too were not poisoned by the food industry that makes them obese-they would have less swelling, inflammation and pain and much more to talk about. Gain clarity about what is truly occurring, reach out to others and gently wake them up.

I unplugged from the gym for over a year now after over twenty years of having memberships for a few reasons: it was a building full of EMFs and, it was an ailment fest, it was depressing. I tried my best to bring knowledge about the chemicals used in a variety of applications at the gym but they were entirely closed to the idea of switching from using toxic chemicals? The chlorine in the pool was so heavy it was dramatically discoloring the swimsuits of the ladies who went to pool class, and I suggested switching from highly toxic cleaners that were detrimental to breathe there was no acknowledgment nor changes made. If you have a gym or other center, or, perhaps you work at a school, begin to bring awareness about detoxification within those environments for the benefit of all.

Unplugging occasionally, and observing what you do with your time, your energy, how and what you eat, what you listen to, even how you spend your money and where you place your attention is giving yourself permission to know and develop yourself. Taking the time to read the book, get yourself a couple composition books one for your plan and your notes and the other for a food diary to get started and then detoxing is **loving yourself enough to heal yourself.** You would be surprised to know how many people resist doing for themselves unless it involves entertainment, or who rarely consider living another way than what they are doing right now. Unplugging means that you spend quality time with you on occasion.

I am not saying that you never again go to the doctor and that you give all that up. I am saying that you have a part in your own wellness. Detoxification is an active part you can do without taking a huge leap, you can begin to bring an awareness about your daily habits, products, food and then move into ways that you can heal your thyroid.

I mean we have well meaning people who believe it is entirely irresponsible to do anything else but be checked by a doctor. With all the fear out there about only trusting the doctor, people have become less inclined to do anything for themselves when it comes to healing, they run right in and get checked immediately. We can detox ourselves and we can consider which food choices may or may not be right for ourselves, and make prudent decisions about lifestyle and products we use everyday. We can introspect and contemplate upon the Mind Body aspects that each of us carries with respect to what shows up for us in relation to our mind and the symbolic physical ways our actions manifest.

Your life is a continuous expression and it is you who must manage it, learn it, love it, and find joy with it. It is you who must learn from many experiences of life. In the world today we 'medicate' and control, we *seek* to cure immediately without pausing for understanding **learning from what is being revealed. The lack of ease globally, is equal to what we see in the body.** We feel scared, humiliated, and we begin to leak energy. Being fearful produces a world energetically that we have created like never before, where we have so many security cameras nearly everywhere: the more we separate, isolate, and produce distrust, the further we will lose our health and our joy.

Part of our medicine is reconnecting with life; it is not just an office visit and a prescription. It is not just another bottle at the health food store promised to take it all away for you.

**Your medicine** is more than just a visit to the natural food store-it is a journey. If you are living a miserable life, whether you acknowledge it or not, you will not produce health. If you do not like your job, your relationships are pained and stressful, and your environment is dangerous and toxic you will not live well. Realize that everything is energy. And, that our thyroid gland health or lack of health, is a **direct reflection** of our state of mind. If you have ever watched the movie, Avatar I know you will see the difference between living in partnership ways and truly caring for the whole vs. living isolated, separate, fending for yourself and fearing your brothers and sisters. **Wounds caused these problems we have today-we must heal them. We can no longer live isolated.**

# CHAPTER SIX - DIAGNOSIS, TREATING, & MEDICATIONS

Most people today schedule an appointment with their doctor to review questions about their health. We want to confide with the person we trust, ideally where we have built a relationship and we know that we can learn something about what is happening with us.

It is almost a given today that we receive testing-most often, blood testing. Ultrasound, CT Scans, MRI and other forms of testing and scanning are tests most people have all had at least once in their lives. If you discuss with your doctor the possibility that you may have thyroid issues, or the doctor has reason to believe that you may, the doctor will order a TSH, or, a thyroid panel, perhaps some adrenal testing and then report back to you if your test was within the normal range. Doctors often palpate your throat to check for swelling and on occasion they will order a thyroid ultrasound to check your thyroid for growths: cysts, nodules or tumors.

There are many options for healing your thyroid, and while the majority of people would prefer testing to feel as if they can definitively know what is going on with their thyroid gland. There are a few other types of testing that may additionally help you.

### Hair Tissue Mineral Analysis-HTMA

Your hair will reveal many insights about your health. With HTMA you get a full printed report showing you just what is happening with your minerals, toxic heavy metals and nutritional profile which is far different from thyroid blood testing. You are supplied with a kit which includes a small hair scale and very clear instructions so that you can take a hair sample. Taking a small amount of your hair closest to your scalp, you send it in to the lab for testing. The printed report reveals many issues which would assist you to accurately correct your health problems, including mineral deficiencies and excesses, as well as detoxifying the body from heavy metals that are identified in the report as well as what to use to aid the body in removing them.

Hair Tissue Mineral Analysis "HTMA," is a great tool. Hair analysis is painless, easy, and, is affordable compared to most medical testing and procedures. You can be retested periodically so that you can check and see if what you are doing is working.

Canine and equine HTMA is also available. I have these services on my website at www.naturallywithkaren.com

HTMA is a good tool for helping with young children diagnosed with ADD/ADHD, Autism Spectrum Disorders, and, ODD (Oppositional Defiant Disorder). HTMA can indicate any heavy metal issues which may be causing problems with health and emotions as well as thyroid issues. Many mothers may not be aware of other options aside from medications. Would you believe that most with ADHD have a copper imbalance and this responds to high doses of food based vitamin C?

**Self Diagnosis Methods**

**Tongue**

Your tongue will tell you a lot about your internal health. I have developed a habit of just taking a look at it several times per week as I brush my teeth and floss. It can be coated, fissured, cracked, red on the tip, spotted, and just about any way, including very fat and even scalloped along the edges. Remember that a thick, fat tongue is likely a hypo thyroid and a red, potentially hot, thin tongue is a fast or hyper thyroid.

Learn to read your tongue in the mirror, and note in your book what you observe. Often when people begin to detox it can get a bit worse for a bit before your digestion clear the mucous, wheat and congestion, just be patient and keep a watch and note what you observe in your book. If your tongue is coated white your stomach is still trying to digest, while fissures and cracks suggest depletion of key nutrients including B vitamins and Vitamin C.

**Blood Pressure**

How many people reading this always had low blood pressure when they went in for a physical exam or a doctor visit? And, we felt pretty good about our health. Maybe it was very low, something like 95/55 or 100/65, and it had always been low. When you have thyroid issues your blood pressure can be low which can indicate a sluggish thyroid or it is called hypotension. A higher than normal blood pressure is often a sign of a fast or hyper thyroid imbalance also called hypertensive.

On your plan that you are putting together be sure to note if you have either low or high blood pressure and if this is consistent or intermittent.

If you have children when you go to their physical exam you will begin to pay more attention to the subtle signs that will give you notice about your child or adult children with just checking their tongue, blood pressure, body temperature, and reflexes. Low scores would mean sluggish thyroid and faster than normal would be hyper thyroid issues most often.

## Basal Body Temperature

One of the best ways to check for thyroid issues is the morning basal body temperature "BBTs" and what you will do is get a digital thermometer and take your morning temperature before you even get up and get moving. It is best to keep the thermometer close to where you sleep and then, record it for at least a week. For women if you are ovulating take one more week as your temperature can change during this time of the month. If you are a full degree below normal, 97.7 or below before you go to the bathroom or anything else, then you have some idea that your thermostat is not working well, that would indicate to me that you have a thyroid imbalance.
Record your BBTs in a composition book so as you heal and add in your iodine you can see your body temperatures will go back up to normal and your "heaters" will come back on and metabolism increases.
Note your blood pressure, any reflex issues, knee, ankle, elbow, joint swelling if you have any, and your BBTs and anything else so that you can reflect on your journey.

## Body Weight/Frame

People who are overweight are often blamed for eating huge amounts of food, but with thyroid issues their metabolism is not functioning well. If they also consume wheat and do not walk, they will be holding on to a lot of excess congestion and body weight. For people who find it very difficult to lose weight, once they give up the wheat and gluten, and then the dairy, and begin to get the detox going they begin to take the weight off pretty easily. More importantly, they gain their energy back and feel so much better and relieve the stresses of carrying all the extra weight on their frames.

One thing about our body weight and frame that just really shocked me was that because thyroid influences our development in so many ways, Women with thyroid issues can have children born with dwarfism or giantism, meaning they are very short in stature or very tall. This is not discussed very often. Considering how often people are not diagnosed or aware of multigenerational thyroid problems we need to make sure that women are informed as to maternal nutrition to prevent these types of outcomes.

Similarly, to obesity the opposite is true, many people are extremely thin with hyperthyroidism, and it becomes hard for them to have an appetite or gain weight. They have lost a lot of muscle and necessary fat. So, I like to get them on healthy fats for their brain like avocados, raw nuts and seeds, fatty fish that is wild caught and onto magnesium glycinate to calm their system down. As soon as possible on a smaller dose of iodine, perhaps 12.5 mg to begin.

### Women's Monthly Moon Cycle

Many women experience a much better monthly cycle when they have detoxed and healed their thyroid. They have more predictable cycles that come on schedule, and they no longer suffer from extremely heavy menstrual flow. With heavy cycles are often clots. All of this is being caused for the same reason that people end up with cysts all over the body and inside the uterus. Once we detox and heal, the body slow down on making fibrin and cysts.

Most women and girls are mineral deficient and toxic.

Every woman needs to know about magnesium, iodine and removing wheat from her diet. Imagine having an easy cycle every single month. With the tools in this book, and doing the detox you will also be healing yourself in many more ways! Detoxify with many of the suggestions in the book and heal with the minerals and vitamin C food based powder. All those chocolate cravings are a craving for magnesium which is found in real chocolate: cacao!

Women today become estrogen heavy and low in progesterone. Progesterone helps the release of thyroid hormone while excess estrogen is responsible for high triglycerides according to Ray Peat, Ph.D.

### Fingernails, Toenails & Skin

People have forgotten how to interpret the many ways their body communicates with them about their mind and their state of health. You can gather so much about your own health with all of these ways I am discussing with you: Your hands, fingers, and your nails on your fingers and toes all tell you something about your health. Decades past we looked at the inherent constitution of a person which was evidenced by the thickness of their earlobes, their skin, their strength and how quickly they bounce back using their own immune system. Your fingers can show signs of inflammation in the joints, they can be swollen, arthritic and calcified, all the way to Rheumatoid Arthritis. Often, people were not picking up on the many ways their body was showing them to pay attention. Through a computer screen with Skype or another face to face application I worked with people asking them questions in consultations to help them to put the pieces together and successfully be able to regenerate their health.

Take a look at your fingernails and toenails. Are they nice and pink? Do you have white moons or a lunula on each finger or toe? That is commonly associated with having sufficient iodine. Most people today are iodine deficient and this is easy enough to fix.

### Eyes, Dark Circles & Shiners

Common to thyroid issues are the dark under eye circles and puffiness. Nobody like puffy eyes and dark circles under the eyes! Most women have concealer and many other cosmetics to cover them up. Ever wonder why we have them in the first place? Thyroid issues certainly cause them, but so does consuming wheat and dairy products. Congestion and missing key nutrients like magnesium, iodine and selenium, as well as sleep will produce them.

Shiners are those really big dark circles that we often see on children as well. Mothers who had nutritional and mineral deficiencies while pregnant can get them and children who develop a more severe form of hypothyroidism

When we are mineral poor and we lack magnesium and iodine we begin to get dark circles under our eyes. This is also the result of eating wheat and gluten, too much sugar and a high grain and starch diet. Instead of just finding a great concealer to use makeup to cover the shiners up, we can detox, remove the wheat, add in the minerals and get some good sleep and sunshine! They will go away.

Edema

Edema which is most commonly fluid retention in your tissues is common with thyroid imbalances but also happens with consuming wheat and dairy as well. For example, I used to have a mark on my legs and ankles where my socks were because of retaining fluid. I know that plenty of other people also suffer from edema as I saw it often working in massage. Fluid retention is common with thyroid issues and it goes away with detoxification. Fluid retention, stagnation and lack of proper circulation that is corrected by detoxification, walking and healing and getting the minerals into the body: magnesium, selenium, iodine and **food based vitamin C** really make a difference.

Edema and fluid retention also occurs in general due to sodium levels in many prescription medications and other items in your diet, including sodium nitrate, MSG, and glutamate, found in soups and prepared foods; another reason I always suggest to prepare your own foods the majority of the time. Pesticides, and fungicides sprayed on commercial fruits, berries and other foods that we can avoid whenever possible. Many of these chemicals that are sprayed on what we eat are very detrimental to our health.

### Thyroid Blood Testing (venous)

There are many tests that your doctor can order, and testing that you can order privately through laboratories like Canary Club, the link is down below. The most common thyroid test given is the "TSH" which stands for Thyroid Stimulating Hormone, made in your pituitary gland. Other common tests are T3 and T4 which are primarily made from iodine. Some of your thyroid hormones must convert, like T4 into T3. Additionally, many doctors take a Thyroid Panel.

https://www.canaryclub.org/basic-thyroid-profile.html

Doctors will tell you if you are inside or outside of the range for each given test.

I felt my symptoms were severe when I was tested and I was told my thyroid was in the normal range as well as many of my clients. I am not a doctor so I shy away from reliance or interpretation of the tests and stay in my lane which is looking at the way the body and mind are speaking about what is being experienced. I am completely open to blood testing I certainly do not have anything negative to say about them, except that they are two different ways of interpreting a situation. My personal way factors and considers BBTs, HTMA, metabolism, and symptoms and the other way considers the blood test more often as an exclusive means to a diagnosis.

I have had many clients over the years who certainly presented with symptoms that are commonly expressed as hyperthyroidism but tested within the range and were not given a diagnosis. Three of my clients whose wife booked them a consultation had tested and received a prescription for Ambien which I recommended magnesium glycinate, removal of wheat, 5HTP and a few other suggestions for one particular man as the first part of the journey was to help you to sleep, and relax his system from anxiety, insomnia, sweating, a hot tongue and problems relating with people that were beginning to cost him. The time on the phone, or in person, or through Skype is relaxing, calm, and I am present to hear what he shares, and to offer some suggestions that truly work. Follow up consults are to go over progress, answer questions and take the next part of the journey until he is feeling much better. I am always agreeable to work in partnership ways with doctor and other practitioners as we all work for the benefit of the client/patient. This way is not a quick fix, it is a journey.

## Thyroid Testing - Original Medicine

In my way, meeting with clients for many years and finding an underlying thyroid imbalance often, I ask clients to record their BBTs so they have some way to be a part of their journey and also to evidence and confirm for themselves. I ask about cold hands and feet, cold intolerance, fibrocystic breasts, and all the other issues they had manifested. I put together a checklist for consults that they could check off as to what they were experiencing.

Getting to know their journey and what they had already been through, many clients had already experienced endometriosis, some had been through breast cancer, uterine cancer, sleep issues, infertility, a buffalo hump, bone issues, pain, obesity, scoliosis, metabolic issues and more.

Most people with thyroid imbalance do a lot of throat clearing. It is so habitual they no longer even realize they are doing it. They also have swallowing difficulties, and people would absolutely never consider that these had anything to do with thyroid imbalance, but, they do. When I am consulting with somebody I am really paying attention with them and I can pick up some of this that the client may have no idea they have these behaviors, so gently note and discuss them so that they are part of a different way of noting thyroid imbalance other than just blood testing. I observe for hair loss, hirsutism, cretinism, giantism, dwarfism, buffalo hump on the back of their neck, bulging eyes, dry eyes, PCOS, memory issues, endometriosis, Parkinson's Disease, and much more!

Different from Western Allopathic Medicine people are not hearing some of the ways I relate about thyroid and iodine from most of their experiences with their primary care physician. Thanks to Dr. Brownstein, M.D., and his wonderful work and education about thyroid and iodine when I consult with clients I can reference a doctor and relate many ways thyroid can manifest into physical symptoms and experiences.

Most often clients were not used to the way of observation and listening as well as "old ways" of how we see health and healing. They have never had the experience of somebody who suggests that they take a personal inventory and set up a plan. It was foreign to change their familiar food habits and The Upper Midwest was perhaps a bit more resistant.

Somebody, and a woman, who suggested they get out to walk, make their juice, and their own food, go shopping at the natural foods store, or the farmer's market. People confided with me that they were intimidated to go to Whole Foods and that they had no clue how to make food. Yet many did! Men got food processors, and people came to my food preparation classes in Whole Foods and while changes like this take a bit of time and energy they are highly beneficial.

Sometimes the way original medicine speaks in plain and simple terms, and the medical industry has its own language and, has a lot of power. The way it is paid for through insurance for many people. The significant trust of the people, as well as allegiance to it. We are thankful for the medical industry even if I am not happy with some aspects of it. Historically, we became obedient to it, and it is now a dominating force in the eyes of the public and what choices we have to heal ourselves.

Without blood testing and with simple observation, after many years now working with people, I can observe a thyroid imbalance almost instantly today, much the same way I can see Crohn's a mile away, simply by observing the skin of the face, the bottoms of the feet, often, cysts, acne, and other problems. When you work together with people, truly hearing their stories, and you help them, research for them, and seek to understand the Mind Body Medicine aspects of their journey you learn a lot. It is Original Medicine because there is not just one answer for every client, it is a journey which truly involves body, mind/emotions and spirit/nature.

I will always be respectful to Western Allopathic medical doctors and yet I can be direct about our way of medicine being very different. Medical schools teach something entirely different and if the person who becomes a Western Allopathic Medical Doctor does not seek further education, communication skills and cross cultural training as well as emotional intelligence they will not evolve into sensing medicine it will be a mechanical medicine and people do not heal with mechanical medicine they heal with sensing medicine from the heart that hears what they truly need.

I observe a person's eyes, I can sense and observe their skin, body and weight, if they came for a table session, I could quickly and easily sense a great deal when they were on the table. As I gave the massage, using my blend of coconut oil and shea butter, I could quickly sense if they had a great deal of cysts, observe hair loss/thinning, eyebrow sparseness, freezing hands and feet, lipomas including, "Buffalo Hump," you can quickly pick up on fast, rapid speech, fidgeting, and the symptoms they speak about will tell me very quickly what is happening.

I have several clients who are morbidly obese and obviously in a great deal of discomfort in sundry ways: sinuses, heart issues, stomach problems, ileostomy, and a few people I have worked on who have had sinus surgery and related with me that it was beyond painful waking up with two large pieces of cotton stuffed up their nose. When we discussed that they would need to give up dairy and wheat they were ready to do anything, but time goes by and they return to it and suffer the consequences.I relate that they likely will never need another sinus surgery if they change their way of life. If you are helping somebody with their thyroid, please remember, you cannot force people, nor get upset about their decisions. I only feel a way about this and it is only difficult for me when it comes to our collective sustainability and how people who purchase and use products that diminish our sustainability cause me to question if they have the right to continue purchasing irresponsibly when it affects the whole?

Original Medicine perspectives on thyroid with my clients are very different from doctors in that I relate that their thyroid imbalance can be much like an energy leak. Most of the time they are needing a detox and healing which would entail a journey of learning about pre-detox, detox and food, detox and lifestyle, and, getting out and walking, getting to sleep with the Moon and not staying up all night, giving up smoking, drinking alcohol and reducing negativity in their lives including reducing the news on TV. I taught about sleeping in a dark room without blue screens and how they will begin to feel better soon.

People with thyroid imbalances often have or had constipation which will be over, as will the sneezing and nose blowing, and the skin will clear up and the thyroid gland will start to "flash" for many people-they will become cold as they begin to heal their thyroid and decongest it and then, they will become warmer. If they are hyperthyroid they will settle down with magnesium and iodine after their detox and be able to cool down and feel much more comfortable in their own skin. They will sleep at night again and not wake up at predictable times in the morning due to liver congestion and they will begin to remember their dreams again soon. Bipolar and even Schizophrenia settle down, with a good plan and this liberates the client from the undue stress of perhaps having to live somewhere other than where they choose to live and have to take medications that could be prevented.

I have given you all the tools you need from starting your journal or composition book and what to notate as well as a website with free recipes that will come to via your email and then we cover in detail how to detox and how to heal including supplements you may want to use and why. Some people do consultations with me or have others around to keep them inspired and motivated, answer questions and important: stay on track!

I wrote this book because so many people asked me to put something into writing so they would have it given all the thyroid problems in the world today. The book is the affordable solution for handling your thyroid issues naturally. This works for people are diligent and organized, who can take a book and do just fine with following the book, and others really need the support.

There is a lot of research online about iodine and anybody can read it. I have read entire books on iodine and I have read most of the articles written by Dr. Flechas, Dr. Barnes and Dr. Brownstein and I feel very comfortable using iodine for therapy for myself and others. Iodine is available online, I am surprised how many people have no idea of what it does or how to use it, and they use extremely small doses of iodine which will not produce the results desired most of the time. I am also very aware that many doctors has a strong reluctance to using it for some reason?

Original Medicine people like myself have the time to take with our clients and discuss how thyroid affects their lives. I have had at least a dozen younger males who had sexual fetishes and other issues that I know had a lot to do with long standing severe hypothyroidism including one man who was meeting up with women from Craig's List ads which nearly ended a long term marriage and caused a lot of stress.

Having a thyroid imbalance can often distort your reality, being lethargic and drained, can make somebody who otherwise would not be selfish, quite unrealistically selfish! It can entirely diminish somebody's sexual drive or libido to a zero! It can create personality issues and if somebody has thyroid issues and extreme mineral deficiencies they can also develop a brain hemispheric dominance like what we see today in our young people who lean towards left brain dominance. Thyroid issues cause a lot of problems for all of us: our coworkers, students, classmates, family members, and in many ways.

I have worked with dozens of men who most definitely had Hyperthyroid issues and were tested repeatedly and told nothing was wrong with them. Often, they had multiple tests and were told they did not have a thyroid imbalance. They could not sleep, had chronic insomnia, racing heart, racing mind, some had migraines, they often appeared very red and flushed or grayed out in energy, some had the burning tongue effect, and they felt an absolute need to self medicate from the intensity of the hyperthyroid that pushed them into using substances they otherwise would not. What concerns me is the push to self medicate and the way thyroid issues when not addressed nor picked up on testing can push deeper into neurological issues down the road. ALS, Parkinson's, Dementia, Alzheimer's, and many others could be prevented.

One man was using opium that he snorted, another man was using Xanax he bought on the streets, I had one client that used alcohol and Advil PM as well as Ambien. Many hyperthyroid clients used daily cannabis, wax, dabbing, and vaping, and edibles.

**Thyroid Medication**

T4 Replacement Singularly

For the majority of people who receive a prescription for medication following a thyroid diagnosis they are treated with Synthroid or the generic equivalent, Levothyroxine.

The problem is that this synthetic thyroid hormone likely does little to actually *heal* your thyroid.

Most people need iodine to help their thyroid and they honestly need a detox and heal program like one found in this book which tells them about each item they need to consider giving up or replacing.

Many people do not realize that medication prescribed for most people with hypothyroidism and autoimmune disorders like Hashimoto's is synthetic T4 hormone. The side effects for this medication used for sluggish thyroid are the exact problems that are faced by somebody who has a fast, hyperthyroidism diagnosis:

- headache;
- sleep problems (insomnia);
- feeling nervous or irritable;
- fever, hot flashes, sweating;
- pounding heartbeats or fluttering in your chest;
- changes in your menstrual periods; or.
- appetite changes, weight changes.

This is very important that you understand that you can do the research for yourself, commercial synthetic thyroid hormone singularly cannot heal you, it can only treat you and you are risking deeper systemic disease by not healing yourself.

This is precisely why I recommend that you detox and actually heal your thyroid. With an HTMA report you can see what toxic heavy metals and mineral deficits are involved. There are also Doctors available at Dr. Brownstein's and other similar types of medical offices which can do the blood testing and interpret them more accurately, together with interviewing you and listening to your symptoms and prescribing the Bioidentical Hormone Replacement Therapy or "BHRT."

Most people who have been under the stress of thyroid imbalance need detoxification, rest, minerals, vitamin C, iodine, walking and real food; they need a reset. If you know yourself and you know that you are not going to do these things or stick with them you will not achieve the results you seek.

Apparently, thyroid medication was in the top three prescribed drugs in our nation which means that we have a lot of people taking thyroid drugs. It seems odd to me to be prescribing drugs for people, when it is so obvious to me, that we need to be making people aware that their blood, tissues, cells, organs and glands are missing iodine, selenium, magnesium, and, that they need a detox. Detoxification from the halogens, wheat, food colorants, food preservatives, body, hair and nail care chemicals and sleeping in front of televisions and in rooms that are not conducive to sleep. People have ingested a lot of programming about a way of life that is not serving them, and it is pretty obvious.

I educate people for decades now about the hazards of the program that is so engrained in nearly every person I have ever worked with, the schools did an excellent job for over a hundred years now for the benefit of the dairy and meat industries. They have implanted the program that we all need calcium and protein from animal products. Even the young teens and adult still look for protein bars, protein shake powder and men and woman including in their 60s and 70s still purchase large jugs of cow dairy pasteurized and homogenized, and packaged in endocrine disrupting plastic jugs. Synthetic Vitamin D is toxic and the constant use of dairy mucous is devastating to our glands. This is not the milk from Aunt Bessie's cows these are mutated bovine with a lot to be concerned about and in any situation we are not suited to drinking bovine mammary gland fluid. I highly suggest you read The Calcium Lie2.

From an Original Medicine perspective, thyroid imbalances respond to detoxification and healing, ideally you obtain an HTMA to determine toxic load and to help guide you with restoration of minerals and elements. After detoxification, supplements that are beneficial are: Tyrosine, Selenium, Magnesium, Iodine and food based Vitamin C powder.

The body will reset itself and find homeostatic balance once it has the tools it needs.

### T3 Replacement

Today, Cytomel is used as a synthetic form of thyroid hormone T3.

### Bioidentical Hormone Replacement

Many people with thyroid imbalance seek out a doctor who works with Bioidentical Hormone Replacement Therapy "BHRT." These hormones more closely resemble your body's own hormones which is why they are called bioidentical. These are often sublingual and are made by several companies. Synthetic hormones do not work so well for people who are "poor convertors of T4 to T3" hormone.

### Thyroid Ultrasound

Thyroid ultrasound is a way to image your thyroid gland. It is done to check for cysts, nodules or tumors which are then measured by the ultrasound technician and later read or interpreted by a doctor. The report is given to your PCP or the endocrinologist you see so that you are informed of the size, and any recommendations with regard to any nodules that may have been found on your thyroid gland. I typically relate with clients who have suffered many years or decades with thyroid imbalance yet have no diagnosis that it may be warranted to seek a thyroid ultrasound to check the status of their thyroid gland.

If cysts, nodules or tumors are found a recommendation will be made by your doctor. At times a needle aspiration is performed to check the cells of or around the nodule. If the doctor feels that you are able to wait and have a recheck you can do a detox and help the body to release out the congestion and heal itself; people often reduce or eliminate thyroid nodules by doing the detox and following the guidelines in the book as fully as possible temporarily until they have resolved their goals.

Radioactive Iodine (RAI) Uptake Testing, Thyroid Ablation & Destruction/Removal

Radioactive Iodine is used today in the medical industry for testing, as well as causing the thyroid gland to become destroyed in whole or in part particularly when there is hyperthyroidism or thyroid cancer.

There are a great many people suffering with hyperthyroid and I wish I could get them to detox and get the minerals and iodine into themselves to reduce and eliminate these problems. Years go by with Anxiety, Insomnia, racing heart and mind, sweating and the medications: sleeping pills, anti anxiety medications, antidepressants and they are not healing they are exacerbating the problems bringing them to a boil is the best description I can provide which leads them into the fire of thyroid destruction too often.

It is unfortunate that many people are resistant and will not listen nor are not flexible enough to embrace something other than medication that takes personal effort. Their body and mind are in a miserable state where eventually, they would almost do anything including self medicating with toxic combinations to quiet their racing thyroid which is most often demanding iodine and fuel in the form of minerals is what it needs: magnesium, selenium, iodine, vitamin C; a plan to detox and reset from the levels of toxins and lack of minerals to keep it going.

I cannot image ever feeling inclined to use this type of a 'test' or procedure? If your thyroid gland did 'uptake' this radioactive iodine **it would mean that you were very deficient in the type of iodine that your thyroid did need.** Consulting with someone who could help you understand how to calm your thyroid and/or autoimmune symptoms, get mineral testing, and detox and balance your thyroid gland, increase the thyroid function will make your life incredibly better! This is similar to saving your gallbladder, or your heart or brain, you would want to do this first. I have spoken with many people who no longer have their thyroid gland and wish they did!

Most people with thyroid imbalance needed detox and healing, not drugs. But when push came to shove, and they had gone far too long without real medicine, and I mean to allow the body to do what it needs to do it needed a detox off the congesting foods that are causing the problems, and it needed healing with a few subtle ways and reinstating minerals, especially iodine to bring the function back up but, because these ways are no longer available for people today in our clinics and hospitals we respond to the urgent or emergency cries when they have gone on too long.

People with hyperthyroid with or without a diagnosis needed detoxification, and then healing including iodine and minerals a long time ago, but nobody told them how to detox their body, and that they needed minerals, especially iodine. They knew they needed sleep, headache relief, and calming of the metabolism issues-most of which are caused by toxic diet, poor habits and mineral deficiencies as well as a need to detox the body.

Sounds like I have this one size fits all shoe for both a slow and a fast thyroid? People have a thyroid and the thyroid needs iodine. Given the amount of halides that we are exposed to today, they interfere with our ability to use iodine and our soils are mineral deficient, particularly in areas like the Midwest which has always been known as a "Goiter Belt," people had a double whammy: exposures to mercury, dioxins and iodine deficiency, in addition to halides: chlorine and fluoride, in the city water for showering, teeth brushing, and often drinking water and food preparation. Bromine in the wheat and baked good which is a dough conditioner as well as many drinks that are now a staple for many younger people. The wheat is definitely a problem as will be all the GMO foods people are eating today.

I have always done my best over the last three decades to gather real medicine and present it in plain and clear English for people to understand that it is far more simple and not difficult at all to bring about real healing and often, curing. It is like it is hard for people to believe because our healing has been made out to be so difficult.

What is very important is I am acutely aware that without iodine our future generations are born less and less intelligent. I did some of my own personal studies on myself using detox, cleansing, minerals, enzymes, vitamins, and I feel pretty confident about how the body responds well when given what it needs. I have cured instances where I was diagnosed of Asthma, Allergies, Endometriosis, Infertility and Ovarian Carcinoma within myself and many people who presented with many different diagnoses.

When you detox, what you are doing is allowing the channels of digestion and elimination to do what they are supposed to do once again and remove toxins from the body. You are giving the body an intended rest in digestion by reducing the hard to digest foods at least temporarily, reducing calories and overeating so that you can relax the body and the mind, adding in walking to move the peristalsis and cause healing to occur at a fast pace with regeneration efforts and you are helping the major organs to recharge more quickly. For example the skin can eliminate more quickly and efficiently. I prefer to use these natural methods than to wonder why people excessively sweat or do not sweat at all? Meaning, by employing the detox protocols that I have in the book and the walking aspects of it will cause the skin to heal, the sweating to heal or to open up and allow sweating to occur. The food based vitamin C is very restorative, and for many people who were self medicating which is common with either hypo or hyper thyroid they can begin to relax these habits and gain comfort in their own skin again, they begin to feel good again and they value any potential "sacrifice" that they seemed to have to make giving up some of those foods for healing in return. **If they again begin to eat those offending foods they will quickly make the connection why they ended up with the thyroid imbalance they had previously**. For the very same reasons some people wake up and choose to go back to sleep on a consciousness level, people often make the same decisions and fall back to sleep with sedating and congesting foods that will drive them predictably back into congestion, stagnation, cysts, nodules and tumors. We cannot force people and the food industry has designed many of these foods to be incredibly addicting. They are found everywhere in every coffee shop, restaurant, buffet, and roadside fast food place as well as upscale restaurants in no short supply.

It is important that you read and understand this book about detoxing and healing before you begin so the you get the most from it and understand what is happening with your body, your mind, the food industry, and common thyroid imbalances, you can then make an informed and logical decision. Any responsible doctor will be more than willing to have you detoxify your own body and institute self discipline to remove toxic and offending substances and foods, and cause your body to upgrade the way it functions.

For example, even with an Ovarian Carcinoma diagnosis I consistently watched my CA125 scores go down with detoxifying on a steady and highly structured plan that I set up for myself in 2009 which I used for about 16 months consecutively 100% until I achieved my goals. My tissues were tested and all, were cancer free!

Most of the time, even with children you can help a great deal by regenerating their health and improving their intelligence, mood and behaviors. Children can take much smaller doses of iodine and minerals and you can also do HTMA to guide with their health as well.

**It is contraindicated to use supplemental iodine if you are on "medications" like Coumadin and Warfarin, that artificially thin your blood. Iodine is known to detoxify your organs, and help your thyroid gland - and help you as an apoptotic, which helps you to remove the negative cells and proliferate positive healthy cells. Cannabis, iodine,**

cacao and many other natural substances are apoptotic and there is a natural fit with the body to utilize them they are in their original form, cleansing, detoxing and upgrading so long as they are not hybridized which is my objection from using cannabis from it's natural "flower" expression of long ago.

When medicine is no longer truly educating people but finding only the quick fix to end the incessant sting of the pain the result is a life that is off balance and to that end, we all suffer.

## Surgical Thyroid Removal

Your doctor may recommend having surgical removal of your thyroid gland for several reasons. It is a common tragedy, that I wish were avoided and, prevented.

Original Medicine would seek to identify issues with thyroid much earlier to prevent radical solutions after disease has been in the body for far too long without attention.

Ideally we would educate our doctors including pediatricians on how to observe and listen so that we pick up on subtle symptoms. To ask and be mindful of the many who encountered harmful exposures to ionizing radiation so that any repair could be made before degeneration became too significant. Ideally we would learn to regenerate thyroid, much earlier with subtle signs of problems and imbalances to prevent radical responses like surgical removal to prolonged states of disease.

I am certainly not stating there is never a place for surgical removal of a thyroid, there is, however, I find that most people do not know how to observe and listen, nor provide the care and maintenance of their body. They cannot accept nor believe such a thing as they have never heard nor seen of it. In much the same way I have acknowledged, I do not know how to fix my house or my car.

There is a place for removal, however, there is a place for regeneration which is not often experienced in Western medicine, unfortunately. When our thyroid gland has inflammation, cysts, nodules, or cancerous cells, there is often potential to minimize inflammation through many ways: supervised fasting is one such way, IV therapy, Ozone therapy to the thyroid is another, and so is nutrient therapy with juice feasting and reducing the body's energy output so that the body can sleep more often and repair itself.

Far too often today we see people "battle" their cancer. They continue to go to work, but pop in for their chemotherapy sessions, and/or radiation sessions. In the same way we observe women also insert a tampon and continue their busy lives during the time of their menses. To regenerate, we need more rest. We need time if we are to regenerate our adrenal glands in our modern and busy world. In order for our body to regenerate our organs, glands, including our thyroid gland, it requires conservation of energy: rest, minimal digestion and elimination which is easier to obtain with consuming a gallon of freshly made and often high green juices per day which is commonly called "Juice Feasting." It is why there are retreat centers in various places in the world where you can have real herbal tea or chai and juice daily as you rest, you stay somewhere relaxing, quiet which is healing compared to many family homes filled with noise, TV, gaming, and EMFs, yet all of our living environments could be much more uncluttered and without as much toxic electronic pollution within their walls: just rid yourself of the TV entirely!

I would choose to surgically remove my thyroid only as a very last resort.

A few of my own close family members have had their thyroid gland removed surgically. It is my opinion that glaring symptoms were left unattended for far too long. I hope this is part of why you are reading this book is to gain clarity of what your body is telling you or your children so that you are on top of this and you redirect, regenerate energy, and way of life towards prevention. Mind Body causatives, cigarette smoking, lifestyle habits, iodine deficiency, magnesium deficiency, exposure to radiation, and a diet full of wheat, dairy, and processed foods were major factors that lead to thyroid toxicity.

The symptoms preceding thyroid removal were fatigue, heat intolerance, hypertension, tremors, weakness, sweating, anxiety, depression and they could be many more out of 300 or more that are commonly associated with thyroid imbalance. Thyroid cancer is not just silent, even if your throat is not aching or you are not experiencing huge growths on or near your neck-you likely covered up symptoms that were alerting you like a check engine light that we quiet and silence when we "treat" them with over the counter solutions. We dismiss them.

The problem we have with compartmentalizing in the medical industry today, is that the hand and the foot do not communicate? Mental health is separate from Gynecology, and, Dermatology separate from Oncology the separation is not organic in nature: we are a whole body. People often use RAI, or, surgically remove their thyroid gland only to die years later from heart disease, and, make no correlation that it had everything to do with their thyroid gland.

Removal of the thyroid gland did not heal the root cause, it only solved the current set of symptoms for the time being.

We need more education about how to know ourselves and heal ourselves, but we do not have that in our education system today. Often, people are angered or saddened that we placed our trust in a medical industry that is ill equipped to help us *prevent* the maladies we end up with, or we were tested, only to send us home pronouncing we are free from thyroid problems pursuant to their testing. Once your thyroid gland is taken out it is life changing, sadly.

I want to emphasize prevention of thyroid issues so that many people can prevent thyroiditis, hypo, hyper, cysts, nodules, autoimmune, and, removal of their thyroid gland. So we can rethink the use of "medications."

## Prevention & Doctoring

I realize that we cannot snap our fingers and bring back our pristine environment, our women as healers as they once were before the advent of the medical industry, and to cause many people to understand prevention, as well as how important detoxification is to our health and the way we are living today.

Doctors, I know you do not have it easy today, and so in loving support of your precious work, I realize you are instructed on what you can and cannot provide with **standard of care** and **health care management** regulations, which instructs you on protocol for treating patients. My role and the role of the Western Allopathic doctor are different, and yet, they are complementary in many ways. They *should* be for the benefit of our World Family.

Elders always taught the medicine, not schools where their business interests run, but Elders and, primarily Women. Women who knew the land, seasons, the herbs, spices, plants, waters, they knew Earth Alchemy and they cared not because they were paid, but because healing was central to future generations. Before someone mentions that due to doctors and hospitals we are saving lives, less children die in childbirth and all of these which I have heard for long years, it simply is not true and what is true is that a progressive removal of our ways was intentionally set into place over thousands of years for a monopoly to ensue as it has today - that, is the truth. Women know how to catch babies, and women know that a common cold is a cleansing opportunity. We just did not "catch" many of the diseases long ago as many of them that we have today were invented, as well as they are part and parcel of our degraded and diminished self, and environment. You see, they are a Message. The Message is that we are not well if we continue to soil our own environment and allow destruction of our ways, means and habitat, our seeds, food, water, air, and the stress on the backs of the people who are forced to pay for life. It's choking us and it is a major factor involved in thyroid disease (lack of ease). It's epidemic and by the way, disease is not evidenced, measurable, nor is it conquerable, neither a battle that must always be won! It is an opportunity to become introspective, to glean the emotional, mind body causatives, to observe the environmental, and to reorganize the physical. It is an opportunity that must be taken within for consideration; it is about life regeneration, not just yours but for those who come after you.

47

Where is our attention taken that we do not prevent? Without necessary minerals we cannot effect increased intelligence, elevated intuitive sensing which is necessary to know yourself and be aware of the subtle ways your mind and body are giving you information.

We must be entirely present and highly ordered in order to unwind, or, "reverse," disease from how it began. The medical industry has entirely abandoned Mind Body Medicine, and what we choices we have out in the world today are mainly guided meditation. Mind Body Medicine is far more than what is most often utilized today; nothing as I have begun to use it in my consultations with clients growing in it's understanding and potential for use for us all. I have progressively grown to understand its enormous potential. Part of this powerful medicine being dismissed becomes expected and, obvious: **it works**, and, the other part is that people were intentionally removed from taking personal responsibility and the power over individual health care was deliberately transferred into the hands of your doctor. If you hear people today, they defend this relatively new position of power of "The Doctor," and, they defense it as they would any other position relative to church and state adamantly. Many systems also have an appeal to people who are very legalistic and who are very concrete in their ways and thinking.

You can easily cause your thyroid gland to heal and, at the same time, you always have the option of hiring the doctor for review, opinion, testing, surgery or anything else you want as long as you pay them or, your insurance does; it is that simple.

Why is massage therapy not covered by insurance? It works too well.

I wish that we had food available for all people, food that was without pesticides, herbicides, fungicides and further, that we had great food forests, clean water, and that we all cleaned up the mess that has been made. Would it be wonderful to have people who have the mindset of healing and regeneration within places people come for healing as a start, that we had people inside of hospitals and clinics that were also "covered" for the majority of people to be able to meet with to gain direction. Clarity about our way of life, prevention and healing will have a large ripple effect for the whole of society improving things for us all.

Along your thyroid journey for detox and healing be mindful please, that you do not allow a general doctor nor anybody else to tell you that your thyroid has absolutely no connection to mental and emotional issues that arise commonly with thyroid gland imbalances, it is one of the top reasons why people feel anxiety, confusion, have memory problems, including intense brain fog, forgetting constantly, migraines, headaches, stomach aches and selfish behavior: people with thyroid issues that are longer lasting feel a very severe shortage of personal resources and end up with many other problems the result of their temperature, immune, heart and brain not working well. It is my aim that we do our best to help people to avert these pitfalls.

**The Many Forms Thyroid Imbalance Take and Why?**

In an ideal world, we would be educated towards self care and self observation, knowing when we are slightly off balance and do subtle improvement immediately to correct the situation and restore homeostasis. Yet with our modern diet, lifestyle and products today we have many problems at the same time, and a lifestyle that is toxic, chaotic and without adequate sleep and rest, too much stress and we are hyper focused on the outside package instead of the integrity, vibration and electricity of the organism. It seems quite juvenile that we decorate our outer house and yet we do no housekeeping for our internal health?

**Cysts**

For years, I would see at last one new client per week at my shop for a massage treatment. People came because they received a massage and often, I related messages, medical intuition, or I saw images which I told them about. But one thing I noticed regularly was cysts, lumps and bumps throughout their clavicle, under their arms, gristle around their hips and bumps around their neck often. Yet, they had no idea whatsoever they even had them?

I have repeatedly suggested in this book, that you are by way of being on this journey and reading this book, becoming your own physician. So that you gain knowledge of self and can heal your self. **We would know ourselves and notice that we are congested and full of cysts.**

When I began offering massage therapy in February of 2003, I observed that nearly everyone coming in had cysts near the breast area and when I would massage near the breast drape and then over the arm and near the armpit I would feel many small bumps and lumps. I felt the "gristle" around and along their hip bones. **I felt how starch stiff their feet were.** Many people had "toenail fungus," which is caused by an unhealthy gut and candida, found often in people who drink alcohol regularly as it is a sugar to the body and feeds the living microorganisms that produce the fungus that love to reside around feet and toenails.

They build nests in the brain and they produce problems including dementia symptoms, memory issues, and brain fog, low energy and skin rashes.

If we knew ourselves we would have noticed the congestion and the cysts-but most had no clue? So, we "feed" them with congesting foods that are not fit for human consumption like dairy products: milk, cheese, sour cream, yogurts, and cottage cheese which congest and congeal the cysts and exponentially cause more problems and now, these cysts become hardened alongside living in a sea of signals (EMFs, wifi, radiation), and they become nodules.

## Feeding The Cysts or, Feeding Your Cells!

People often wonder how it is that they have tumors? Where did they come from? How did they get there? They wonder how long have they been there, and, why is it I did not find out until it was "too late?" I have my thoughts about our lack of ease and I find a pretty simple analogy, I am amazed at how complex people make it out to be and often, people do not feel like they can trust how truly simple it is.

## The Five Key Principles:

1.  Your body is water and minerals, most of us do not have sufficient mineral balance
2.  You need very little in the way of food and most if not all of it is plant based
3.  You need sleep at night
4.  You need exercise and time in Nature
5.  You need a life with far less stress


1.  You are water and minerals and yet most of us do not have real water, I mean the breast milk of Mother Earth. The human nipple and body supplies instant nutrients, minerals and antibodies and so does our natural spring water which gathers precious minerals over the rocks, but, you may remember, that with Hoover, we began to dam our water and re-direct it's flow, we began to "treat" our water and now it is piped through corrosive, formerly lead and often copper pipes, leading to contaminants, excess metals, minerals and problems. We need real water and that means we have to get back into taking care of this precious aspect of life, necessary for all. Today, we are spinning our wheels distilling, alkalizing, and purifying water when it was formerly unnecessary.

We are all deficient in key minerals like iodine, selenium and certainly magnesium, often we are deficient in copper and sometimes people have copper excesses. Lead was found in Michigan and there is a lot more that is not reported because when we have a centralized government we fail to have the type of guidance that we would have in Elder Councils that were making sure people, the land and all beings were living in accordance with natural law, the most visible and common sense approach to life is, sustainability and harmony.

2.     People are overeating for several reasons, and because they are missing key minerals. Let's take wheat for example: it was specifically bred to become what it is today and, it is everywhere under the guise that it was *bred* for helping an explosive population cope with food demands and farmers needing to make a profit. However, in the same way we have unnatural agriculture, landscape, plants introduced into areas that are not copacetic, we have people occupying concrete jungles, we have far too many linear, box and commercialized ways of looking at life. How we must see food now, what food is, and how it is created as it has become "frankenfoods," directly destructive to you and the environment. The pesticides, fungicides and herbicides have caused many problems. These are our problems and, it is irresponsible to leave them behind for future generations to deal with, our children and forward generations must deal with these atrocities now.

People overeat today, plain and simple and, this directly affects your throat, your thyroid gland and your gut, all of which must be detoxed and you must get enough minerals or you instinctively begin to root around and eat more in an attempt to gain those minerals.

3.     People need sleep, and many do not know that they need it at night, "with the Moon." Meaning that ideally when it gets dark or soon after, we get to sleep. And, we rise with the Sun this is Circadian Rhythm and if you violate it long enough you rob yourself of vital energy and you prematurely age. Yet in a modern system, we work the "graveyard" shift, and it's 'ok' for a bit, but we end up with foul moods, perhaps even severe moods when we are seriously depleted. Without sleep people are more prone to drug addiction, pain, relationship problems, and without sufficient magnesium in the body the body is tense so sleep is more elusive. With congestion from the foods I mention that you must detox from in order to heal your thyroid you will have not only anxiety, pain, but also sleep problems that are related to congestive sleep apnea. There is no reason for the anxiety, pain and lost sleep, overweight body, rough skin, and the resultant thyroid gland problems. It's not difficult to detox and heal your thyroid. I became so fatigued mentally with providing massage therapy for people who had bodies like a cow, they were toxic because of their social eating habits-they refused to change. And, since their doctor did not verify thyroid disease and place them on a synthetic thyroid hormone they were going to carry on with digging their graves with their teeth and habits.

4.     Exercise is something most people would really benefit from in a big way. I mean they go to gyms and have a social visit, they clean their homes, and organize and do sitting projects like quilting, knitting, and a bit of gardening, and yard clearing on occasion but then, they cannot bend down and touch their own toes. They do not walk in Nature each day. They

are overwhelmed and they never put in place these daily habits. If you ask them about their flexibility and you speak about how flexibility of the spine equals flexibility of the mind, often they agree with you but they just won't do it? They eat pasta, factory farmed chicken, cheese, fried eggs, bacon and they do not realize what they are doing and how they are spending their money.

People need real exercise, not strenuous exercise, but they need at the very least an hour out in Nature every single day absorbing the sunlight, the plant energy - It is the sunlight condensed into the plant life and the fresh morning dew on the leaves that is respirating into the air as you walk amongst the plant life and the trees and in the winter the fresh crisp air, the crunch of the snow, or near the negative ions of moving water, or the ocean waves, all of which release the mind, and the reflex points on the feet. We are geared to be foraging and gardening for our foods, preparing simple foods, not frying, excessively cooking our foods, but simple easy to eat foods that grow in nature and now, we are consuming grains that are processed into "pasta," or paste, and walking less and less. Nature, whose symbol is the Wolf has become "scary" the Forest is just what is states, it is for rest for you, it could be again our safe place, the place we go to heal and rejuvenate except that with the industries I speak about in this book, things are out of balance and that has us throttled by the neck and our thyroid gland showing us the Mind Body aspects of our humiliation, as well as with physically, clearing our throats, we see more and more people hocking up a loogie all over the streets, mucous laying about, hearing it being brought up from the throat, and anxious people, competing for resources and living as if life for our forward generations is without promise? That daily habit of getting outside each and every day to the extent possible and absorbing the beauty the life, the fresh air, the oxygen, increasing our blood flow, releasing the tension of our mind is vital and crucial.

5.      Stress is ugly, right? It's cramming for tests to get through academia so that you can work more, or earn more money, so that you can race home and have enough time to heat up your food and run back to work, so that you can get to the bank before they close and get your check in and all of it is not only unreal it's harmful! I lived it for years and the largest stress I ever had was surrendering my only child to stranger care (daycare), ever! I now scratch my head and wonder how it is that we all complied with this insanity? I see more mood disorders, raging, like I once did with my thyroid being so out of order, and my adrenals being so exhausted, I understand the HPA Axis of my mind and my adrenals and how they pumped and pumped to keep me going. How the Pavlovian good dog kept seeking strokes to feel as though I was doing "good." But it was all backwards, clearly it is - we are not getting better and we are not getting healthier, our relationships in general are not better, there are strides here and there, but

not terrific progress and we need that before we cause even more self and planetary destruction. Stress is the one aspect of life that causes mental tension which decreases blood and oxygen flow to the tissues, and muscles and it will cause you certain distress with your thyroid gland. Your thyroid also does not care if it is positive nor negative stress, it cares that you tone it down and adapt to life by using these tools like the ones mentioned above with walking in Nature every day. Ever notice how many people around you have the pug dog looking bulging eyes? We call that "Graves Disease." We have a neat container for each and every collection of symptoms, however, it is when the eye became dry, the area around the eye orbit became inflamed, because it should make sense that you thyroid is in your throat and it when it is inflamed will cause pressure on not only directly your ears which will have ringing and buzzing perhaps, or, "tinnitus," but also your eyes! You often get dry eye but you also get bulging eyes because the eyeballs themselves will protrude from the orbit of the eye due to the systemic inflammation.

When you detox and you continue to eat eggs (histamines), factory farmed meat, nitrates, white sugar and white salts, artificial spices and foods with MSG, or glutamates, disguised as natural flavors often, you inflame your body

I love people, yet often when I tried to listen to good people in their live streams it was difficult to be entrained with their messages when you are hearing rapid speech, and mesmerized by their bulging eyes and add insult to injury and they are sipping on their "morning coffee with creamers" which I see as "jacked up," on chemicals and caffeine, eating their morning toast, (wheat), the body looks dry, lackluster, the hair is dyed, having been chemically colored and the face is painted up, the fingernails are painted up and they have no clue what they have done to themselves? Just trying to educate about how obvious it is to me that they are entering a danger and artificial zone. The doctor has not diagnosed them *yet* just like many of my clients who already had their breasts removed, and far too many symptoms which seemed obvious to me originated in their thyroid gland. You must be sick and tired of doing the same thing and getting the same results. Yet, I have learned people get offended because they feel attacked, even when you "feed" them the truth-of course it hurts, of course it's painful and of course, you will have to learn new ways as the ways you are accustomed to are not working and will produce exactly what you are steering yourself towards: cell death.

I hope you see that we have forgotten, and what is waiting for us is real life again, one that is not dependent upon the systems in place that are profiting from our removal of knowing ourselves and being real again. We systematically became reduced by seduction. Seduced into formula being better, into smelling better, into a product that helped us to not have to iron our clothing, like dryer sheets, or soften and smell up our laundry, and products that helped us to not have to stink when we deposited foods into our bodies that would cause it to stink. Over the counter products that reduced the mucous for us so we could continue to deposit the mucous in the form of a plastic endocrine disrupting jug of cow pus that is so manipulated over decades now these poor beings are hardly even anything similar to an original cow?

Our endocrine system is your hormonal system and what your thyroid is doing is pumping your hormones, and making thyroid hormones which is its job, it cannot do its job if you do not do the 5 key things I have listed above. You will make cysts and your body will prepare to shut down, for some people that will be soon and for others that will be decades from now, depending upon how much abuse you have done to yourself and your family habits and patterns. What I know for a fact is that multi-generational issues are different from heredity and genetics exclusively, they are the habits your family has about control, aggression, privilege, perfectionism, daily life, getting outside and walking, relaxing, pushing back on stress, how you eat.

Is your family still using a BBQ and eating hot dogs? Are they stocking up on 2-3 jugs of cow milk per week and bacon, eggs, making hash browns, and starching, mucous, and denatured foods are big part of their daily movement? Well, then social habits have to change, or, you can predict and expect situations like Alzheimer's Disease which is just over 40 years in the making now to come to you, Dementia, and the host of neurological diseases that are not random. Often then come from parasites hidden in your spine, your brain, your colon because you kept feeding them cyst making foods and you did not supply the iodine and other minerals to keep your body homeostatic.

Watch the people who are afraid to make simple and necessary changes challenge what I am saying they need to find fault so that they have an excuse not to do what will help them to detox and heal their own thyroid. You see I realize now thirty plus years in that certain people will adamantly and staunchly defend staying married to their diagnosis, or their demise to the very end and those are not the people I can help, neither can you, sadly. They are in my own family and they refuse to make simple, easy and effective changes that will not even cost much? Watching them die day by day is beyond painful, but eventually you must just do what you can do to be a "Model Worthy of Imitation." That is what the Bible is truly all about is guiding people through modeling behavior and habits that are worthy of imitation or repeating by the Youngers from the Elders. It's just beyond sad that people go through 12 years of learning their own Mother tongue: English, bogus history most of the time, and they are completely removed from home and hearth which is why I valued the Waldorf Schools so much, because of their appreciation and knowledge about maintaining the imagination-without it you end up with automatons and people with no sense of imagination, they are like the helpless cattle of today, only listening to the doctor and not their own common sense. They were never taught to listen to their own body, to read their own tongue, pulse, heartbeat, and so they are held hostage by a system which will never prevent what they will "get," it will exacerbate problems with drugs that are overlay their conditions to assuage their symptoms.

All that you ever need is already here, but, will we preserve it and increase it for all of our future generations? Or, will we deplete and destroy it and continue to hand our teenagers sleeping "medications," anxiety "medications," antidepressants because they genuinely pick up on the problems presented so obviously and clearly in the world? Will we drug ourselves to death? I said that blood thinners are a racket because they deplete the body of potassium, much like many of the statin drugs that many Elders are convinced that they need.

Your food, your lifestyle, your movement is going to be reflected in your health. Detox, heal and upgrade yourself consistently and you will enjoy life much more. Now, if we could get our children to do this as young adults so that we have vital and loving time together, despite what school systems fed and educated them we would have half the issues resolved. Our children were fed the equivalent of government surplus high fat, toxic food and they now have been drugged like never before or will get their anxiety from their thyroid gland imbalances comforted by a pain medication following a surgery and they will want that feeling again. Opiates were created with this in mind, they have a high potential to addict, they know this and so do you.

Continue to feed the cysts now and they become nodules and then, later, you have diseased tumors. Most of which have been hanging around for many years or decades, waiting for the opportunity to begin feeding upon you as you enter entropy-gradual disorder; no power to fund yourself, you begin to show symptoms for sure by this point that you will pay attention to, and, will be diagnosed as your white blood cell count will "evidence," your demise.

Iodine has shown promising benefits in clearing the congestion from the body, but, you have to be willing to install new habits, willing to embrace change if you are a person who is pretty attached to the mainstream Standard American Diet, and is used to a diet of wheat toast, jars of jelly, cereals out of the box, white salt, pork chops, ham, and ice cream, pies with shortening and flour and eggs on the weekends with fried brown potatoes, you will have to be willing to embrace eating to feed your cells, and eating to live, seeing your food as your medicine not just what is sugary and pleasing and familiar to your palate. This takes courage but it's not only easy to do its fun! I did not give up cheesecake, cookies, cake, pies, lasagna, burgers or anything else, I gave up that which no longer serves me and found ways to enjoy all those things and, feel good after I ate them! So, please, do not worry that you would have to eat truly distasteful things, I wouldn't do that to you!

Thank you Dr. Brownstein for the many teachings and the crucial knowledge of the cyst, nodule and tumor pathway.

### Apoptotics & Neural Communication

Many people are just learning about apoptotic function and how certain plants have the capacity to help us push out negative cells and proliferate positive cells and this is also true for your thyroid gland using certain types of plants as food. But not just what you may think. You see, we often hear about Cannabis and how people use it in many forms, probably the one most celebrated for medicine is the freshly prepared juice. Dark green leafy plants hold on to sunlight and many minerals due to their deep pigment. Their deep pigment contains minerals and also cacao. These two powerful plant based ingredients can really increase your healing exponentially.

Not everyone has the ability to legally use cannabis as freshly prepared and *non-heated* juice, however, obtaining the raw organic leaves is not something I can do at this time, but perhaps where you are located you can? I am including this in the hopes that you can utilize making fresh cannabis juice. Most people I have followed have had remarkable success using fresh cannabis juice and I hope to be able to legally one day soon enough in the state of Minnesota a my grandparents did back in the early 1900s in Pine County, Minnesota. My Grandmother spoke often of how cannabis grew wild and they often made sun tea from it.

What many people do is juice about a dozen or more fresh organic whole leaves and a few buds that are fresh and raw and they note and people mix in apples, carrots, or other fresh fruits or vegetables to make it taste appealing. One thing I know about cannabis is that it is a flower and they are communicators. We know that our cells communicate and that especially nerves communicate so for people who are healing in this case your thyroid it promotes communication. I want to make a something crystal clear here:

Your thyroid gland located in your neck which is connected to your eyes, ears, voice, and often first symptoms of it becoming unbalanced is hoarseness, throat clearing, puffy tissues in the face, and other symptoms include bulging eyes, ear ringing and more proneness to being stuck as thyroid is about feeling heard with your voice and feeling valued with your voice and say in the world. **Cannabis is a communicator, it is a flower** and it facilitates call and response, in our nervous system, our blood and our energy pathways and meridians.

We had everything we needed for vibrant health here on Earth at one time and as we became seduced to sell to one another-we lost much of this due to greed. Greed has kept the majority of us from obtaining absolute luminosity. Luminosity is when you are radiant, fully sensing, detoxed and plant based. We just do not see this today, but at one time people could obtain this level and you see the many reminders if you truly observe. People standing in many powerful structures that are left behind for you to see and with images of our pineal gland and how they are organs and glands that help you to vibrate because you are energy. If your thyroid cannot do the most basic of design, which is to maintain your body blood pressure, cooling and heating, your weight and metabolism your energy will not be strong enough to cause you to become luminous. I have had a few experiences with detoxification and balancing energy. Becoming luminous extends your field outside of the traditional ways of perceiving. You need your thyroid gland to function well and so the purpose of this book is to give you insight about how to detoxify and heal your thyroid gland.

Cacao or cocoa powder is easy enough to use by mixing with clean filtered or distilled water and some coconut palm sugar or the sweetener of your choosing. You could also add a seed or nut milk that you make yourself in your blender with raw seeds or nuts and water, perhaps a pinch of good quality salt. Cacao smoothies and many other ways to utilize cacao for health and enjoyment. To detox and heal your thyroid does not have to be painstakingly difficult nor do you have to deny yourself the enjoyment of taste and good food and drinks, you just have to learn a new way if this way is foreign to you at this time. It is not difficult. Being excited about this new journey is a plus!

We can have some fun using apoptotics that provide nutrients and help the body to discharge negative cells. You can seek out more information about this independently as well!

Many great men have given us stellar examples: Aris Latham, Dr. Sebi and Arnold Ehret all have great messages and wonderful medicine.

### Mineral Deficient Examples

With thyroid problems you will likely visit the chiropractor more often as your neck can come into needing adjustments. Mineral deficiency causes a lot of problems. Learning disabilities, cancer, sinus issues, organ toxicity, but also cyst growth.

Because they ran of of minerals necessary to build bone, fund their brain, make hormones, digest, run their elimination and most importantly, their central nervous system. Without minerals you cannot make connective tissue, myelin for your nerves and this is precisely why some people suffer from Rheumatoid arthritis, colon cancer and others get diagnosed with Parkinson's Disease, or Multiple Sclerosis. Too many women end up with breast cancer and not just because they have a genetic mutation on their breast, because their breast needs iodine to maintain health.

People have reversed breast cancer with high levels of iodine, diet, lifestyle, exercise sleep, amino acids, minerals. Can you imagine the polar opposites: as opposed to how we handle breast removal in the hospitals. I encourage you to check into this for yourself.

Thyroid glands are inflamed, swollen, slowed down, diseased for obvious reasons. This book is not intended to diagnose, "treat," nor prescribe that is not my domain. It is about detoxification of your body so that it can do what it is geared to do-maintain homeostasis and work well consistently and for long years with subtle corrections and adjustments, plenty of walking, good sleep, and real, nutrition, high plant based, enzyme and mineral rich, with good quality mineral rich drinking water.

People are very habit-orientated, they will continue doing what they do just because it is what they do. For example, once we have done something during our childhood days, often we will continue as a habit even if it clearly does not work. In order to form daily habits of self love and become successful, you will have to write down a plan for yourself and then make sure you do it the first few times so that you feel a comfort with a new daily habit until you grow into familiarity with caring for yourself.

For example, I most often encounter people who are mineral deficient. In order to find that mental calm and balance, I want for them to first, take a probiotic to begin healing what is far too common today, digestive distress, leaky gut and and inability to procure nutrients from food. I realize that beginning with simple habits will create a new program for most of us to love and care for ourselves where we may have just started our day with turning on the news on the TV and dishing up negativity, which is also a kind of food and affects us mentally and energetically, and then we head out the door to find food, often the kind of food that we grab and get to work with, often something inexpensive and yet very destructive. A warm sandwich that is financially inexpensive and we do not have to prepare anything because we feel too busy and without enough time to prepare something, nor do we want the mess of preparing it in addition to feeling as though we do not have the time. Convenience is an illusion when it comes to these grab and go foods, energy drinks, bags of GMO pretzels, chips, plastic containers of iced tea with lemon, chewing gum, and the variety of bars that allegedly are healthy for us. They appeal to our tongue because they are highly addictive and why? Because they are wheat, gluten, plastic, sugar, and they are not only addictive they are highly destructive; they will take a huge toll on your health.

Each morning I have you take a probiotic which is easy to do when you write it down and set your plan down on your table, counter, near your bed or anywhere else you will see it. Set positive messages around your home that are contrary to what you see and hear often in the common programming, for example, I have a beautiful small wooden sign from the dollar store that says, "Believe in Yourself." I will post colorful index cards in a few places with a pleasant affirmation or something written that I want or need to do in my life to get to my next goal, if you do this you will be more successful.

You could write down Probiotic in the morning and Magnesium in the evening an hour or so before you prepare to wind down and go to sleep. You could write down on a card to minimize or better yet remove the "news" from your life so that you hear what you hear from people around you but not necessarily a steady "stream" of sensationalized negativity all the time. When we heal our thyroid gland, we are restoring balance to our central branch of government in our body that which lies between the head, the brain, like the mainframe computer and the body like the vehicle. Fear, sadness, grief, humiliation, a sense of being choked out of life is something we all see on the news today and something we must learn to avoid heaping doses of, especially as we first rise in the morning when we could be taking a few moments to get our probiotic, cut up some melon and make ourselves a delicious blended drink to take out the door with us and begin our day fresh, nourished and thankful!

After our day, be sure to have your evening habit, your magnesium glycinate near your bathroom, or bedroom near your sleeping area, or somewhere you are absolutely sure to see it, and a small sign, post it note or something to remind you to initiate these new daily habits of self love and success. Magnesium Glycinate will begin to relax your central nervous system and feed your body minerals to aid in many ways, including sleeping and waking more rested, restoring your glands and for purposes of detoxing and healing your thyroid gland, it will also aid in your adrenal gland function which becomes depleted for most of us keeping up with the pace of the world today. Before I suggest what would overwhelm most people we begin simply with easy to do new habits and once they become habits and people feel so much better they are more relaxed, they find it quite easy to implement the other daily habits until they are a solid way of life and you are free from the burdens of most imbalances in your body and your health. Once you are sleeping better, your gut is digesting better, you are more relaxed and less anxious, more present, you take the time to write down your plan out of what I provide for you in this book you can achieve goals easily and simply.

Now, you can prepare to detox in a few short and easy ways and once you feel that comfort you can proceed into learning about your food, your lifestyle and products, and you will experience that a way of life is more important than just medicating yourself and expecting profound results from a pill alone. Often, it may take a combination of making sure you are comfortable each step as many of my clients did they continued to check in with their doctors and their doctors were extremely surprised at how they were actually healing from issues that they were told would not heal. Of course we heal, it is our nature. You must believe you heal, understand your body and what it needs on a very basic level and be able to tune in to yourself and know what habits you can set up for yourself that will bring you results!

### Thyroid Imbalance & Suicide

We have more suicides of adults and young people happening in the world and sometimes even on social media sadly. I know how miserable you can feel with thyroid and autoimmune issues, and, helping somebody to pull up and get their spirit back is not something you just fix overnight, but, there are a few ways I am aware of that can make a difference. Getting the person to take some Magnesium Glycinate as well as 5HTP are both mineral and amino acid which helps to calm and restore the spirit as well as a good cup of tea, some lavender essential oil and bit of positive energy from people who care about them. If you are having feelings of suicide, please know that you can get through this and you can honestly and wholeheartedly feel so much better so quickly that you will won't believe you ever felt this way when you look back!

The lack of minerals and the need for removing toxic load are why people are feeling this way. In the same way that we all can smell under our arms when we eat something that does not agree with us, or it smells when we have a bowel movement, you have an accumulation inside of you that is being felt in another way, it is poisoning your spirit and your mood. I can help you if you work through the book and turn things around for the positive! I'm with you!

Once you get through the first day or two and begin to turn things from a low mood into a higher mood, set up your plan and make sure you take the magnesium gycinate every night, and start with about 3-10 mg of vitamin c, food based if possible and your 1 tablet of 5HTP early or late morning some time after you get up in the morning.

| | |
|---|---|
| 2 | Magnesium Glycinate @ night |
| 1 | 5-HTP @ morning |
| 1 | Vitamin C (food based) 1 gram- 3 times day |

Now you can begin to detox and feel results within one week. When somebody is low, chances are their minerals are low. They are not funded with energy and they begin to think negative and low grade thoughts.

Once you get some detoxing done and your vitamin C levels up to 1 gram 3 times per day you can then usually begin using iodine no problem. The iodine will also thin the blood, detox your organs and bring relief in many ways. Dr. Brownstein mentions in his book, Iodine, Why You Need It, 5th Edition (2014), that:

"Iodine intake in daily amounts from 50 to 75 mg iodine in the form of Lugol's tablet (Iodoral®) had a positive effect on the saliva/serum iodide ratio and decreased serum bromide."

**For somebody just starting out-12.5 mg of Iodoral and then transi-**

**tion into the higher doses as you feel comfortable.**

I have family members who committed suicide. My paternal uncle Don Pringle for one, and I know from experiencing several people who became suicidal that when your thyroid is not well, you can feel pretty low. Most people cannot take the continuous gnaw at your mind and some are as stubborn as it gets they refuse to start helping their own body to reduce the toxins, cysts and start healing as they deny that minerals and food will do anything but they are miserable with insomnia, anxiety and even addiction? As we get more clear on our ways of detoxification, we are also ridding ourselves of parasites. Parasites occupy a host and then they do what? They feed upon it.

For anyone who may be reading this right now who has recently or ever felt suicidal: we want you here! There is help if you set up a plan for yourself and follow the book or get consults immediately and get to rebalancing.

# CHAPTER SEVEN - PREPARING TO DETOX

How exciting, I want to make sure that we discuss some pre-detox:
Make sure that you now have the composition book or journal, and, a food diary. These are easy enough to pick up 2 compositions books or more at the dollar store for about $2. Let's make sure you answer the first three questions in your book, write them down and then answer each of the three please:

1.    You are eliminating well-having bowel movements once per day easily
2.    You have reasonable digestive function and can handle plant based food
3.    You write down your current weight, blood pressure and any diagnosis or symptoms

One of the ways I encourage to get going first, is to begin by purchasing just 3 things. Write down in your journal any of these steps you will be taking on the Pre-Detox page:

1.    **Skin Brush:** A wooden handle natural bristle skin brush. Keep it handy where you will see it and use it!

**Directions:** Use it dry only, and use small strokes towards the heart on your dry skin before or after showering or bathing, or, in addition to sponge bathing always in the direction of your heart. Start at your feet by bending and, breathing and with your brush in hand and using small flicks of the wrist, come up from the toes, tops of the feet, fronts of the legs, knees, front of your thighs and into the corners of your pelvic region, softly up the belly, and softly around the breasts, under the arms downward now towards the heart and a tiny bit if you wish on the throat that houses our thyroid gland. Because some areas of your body have more sensitive thin skin, go a bit lighter in pressure-you decide where and how you will use it. You are not only detoxing with this daily habit, which is now free after the purchase of the brush, it takes only minutes, and, also beautifies your skin, moves your lymph and uplifts your mood in just a minute or two.

Duration:    Daily, time: 1 minute

2.    **Probiotic:** this is part of a detox because it is helpful to rid microorganisms like candida, clean up the gut by depositing beneficial bacteria and help with better digestion and elimination.

**Directions:** Shop around at natural food stores and find a good quality probiotic in the refrigerator section that has many strains of bacteria and potency. Prices range from $5.95 for a single strain acidophilus all the way to $60 or more for a stronger probiotic. Keep it cold and refrigerated or you can also opt for the type that is enteric coated which means it will make it down to your stomach to be utilized with a special coating and does not need to be refrigerated. Take one first thing in the morning with room temperature filtered water. It is important to note with probiotics that you rotate your strains; when you select your next bottle select a probiotic with different strains of bacteria and strength so that you are not depositing the same bacteria month after month and you keep your body out of a rut. I thank Joe Meese, the Compounding Pharmacist formerly of Prescription Specialities in Duluth, MN for his great insight on the rotation aspect of probiotics. Now, if you have a leaky gut, or, a lot of gut issues, also called your "microbiome" today, you could safely take a probiotic two or three times per day to increase gut healing.

Duration:    Daily, time: 1 minute

3.    **Clay and/or Diatomaceous Earth** will definitely come in handy! Both for oral, hygiene    and supplement uses. Cost is about $5-$20

**Directions:** You can find food grade clays, like Bentonite or Redmond Clay that can be taken internally, and, which act as detoxifiers as they pull toxins and help to excrete them through the bowels as well as provide Earth element minerals. Nice thing about clay and, Diatomaceous Earth also known as "DE," is that both tend towards pulling out excess radiation, parasites, especially the simple pin worms which will be reduced or removed first through the bowel movements-we pick them up everywhere. Diatomaceous Earth "DE" are diatoms from the sea floor so this is a bit different from Earthen clay like Bentonite and Redmond Clay that is food grade. **DE is purported to assist with pulling out radiation from the body** and I use it with my clients to restore the gut, help with parasites, and also, to help those nail bed ridges on our finger and toenails. Friends from childhood related that just using DE with water in the morning trimmed their waistline, and helped them have regular bowel movements.

Of course, if you are on any medication please take a moment and review if this is going to be alright for you to begin a gentle form of detox. Most of the time, there is no problem with probiotic, skin brushing, nor clay or DE, however, it's best to ask your doctor especially if you are taking medications. DE is sold in a bag with a texture technically like a "flour," and part of how it works is that it can grab parasites-it has barbs which are microscopic. Make a plan not to open the bag and smell it after shaking it around, as it could irritate you a bit and it should say on the bag that open it away from your nose if it's been moving around in the bag as it is a flour. By the way, you can brush your teeth using clay or DE and, you can make a facial or even a gentle acne scrub for your face or body with DE or the clay, and, if you have blackheads you can add a bit of apple cider vinegar.

**NOTE: when using Earthen clay or DE, do not use METAL implements like spoons, or to mix, use wooden, bamboo, silicon, clay, or glass bowls. A good use for recycled chopsticks.**


I find that if most people do too much too fast they tend to feel overwhelmed especially with thyroid issues. So, depending upon your age, your physical shape and what you have going on with medications, or any stomach issues take this at a comfortable pace and it is your custom plan to detox & heal your thyroid gland. You do not have to do everything I suggest, there are plenty of suggestions that you can choose the ones that work well for you and definitely do not have to do them all.

We are setting the stage so that your body can begin to transform. So that we can get your thyroid gland balanced and well, first let's read through the book and note what you want to do and in what order so that you can get any supplies that make the best sense given what you know about your thyroid and body. In this way, we are taking good care of you and making sure that you can easily release toxins from your body which will begin to heal your thyroid.

Use a page of your Composition Book or Journal that says: **Items to be purchased and write down the following:**

Probiotic
Skin Brush

Bentonite Clay/Redmond Clay/DE (Diatomaceous Earth)

You could get all 3 for under $25 and you could also spend more.

In my experience, I have found that often, people are not entirely comfortable taking about their bowel movements, I mean who would right? So, if you are eliminating every single day and it is a brown log, not too big and consistently you eliminate this way every day, you are probably fine to do the first basics of detoxing-preparing the elimination.

Lastly, I want you to spend some one-on-one time with your thyroid-sounds kind of odd right? But, here's what it looks like: stand in front of a mirror and take a look at your neck, take your fingers and stroke the skin at the base of your neck and feel for any lumps, bumps, small rashes, take a minute or two and feel your neck and look into the mirror, notice what you feel first, and then, what you see, and, how you react.

This is important and you may be tempted to skip this step but please, do it and write down what you feel, see, and, how you react those 3 things in your composition book.

Next, take a washcloth with warm water and gently wash your neck where your thyroid gland is located. I often see massage clients who have bumpy rashes all along the base of their neck and we seem to avoid noticing them, touching, washing or caring for this area of our body? I felt the same way for myself for many years, I hardly touched this area of my body. You are liberating the skin here so that it can breathe and heal from the outside in. Use some gentle soap, or even a mild scrub, or make an Epsom salt scrub to use just for this. You will have to trust me on this and spend this time for a minute or two or five, each morning or evening or whatever time works best for you and give, loving attention to your neck and your thyroid. I want you to send loving energy and kindness to this powerful part of you, and, your thyroid gland, also to hold the intention that you heal. You heal, and not just treat. Medicine, can be far more subtle than you may ever imagine. You, hold the key to your own cells-your own self.

The neck is a vulnerable part of our body. Many people have trauma issues and this can be very powerful work in the present lifetime and ancestrally. The neck is very symbolic and was involved in hangings, and all sorts of trauma, and represents being choked off from life. We are placing our intention for life upon our neck, throat and thyroid. Do this for a few days or make it a habit that you spend another 1 or more minutes upon and do write it down in your composition book, please.

Other Pre-Detox Ideas

If you have the interest, the time and the cash, you could do this basic cleanse for 3, 7 or 14 days which goes quickly and you can pick one up online through RenewLife.com.

You could also get a *Basic Cleanse* for about $29 and works really well and, is simple enough to take herbal capsules in the am and pm. Just review the contents and make sure that you are healthy enough to do this and clear your elimination first. Renew Life has a 3, 7 and 14 day as well as a *First Cleanse* for older adults like myself who have never done a cleanse. I have enjoyed and, trust their products for nearly 20 years now professionally. I have had a good experience learning from the company, and getting good service from their customer support.

The goal here is to get your gut healthy, your skin detoxing and moving lymph and blood, removing toxins and get your elimination channels going well.

Let's move onto Detoxification & Food!

# CHAPTER EIGHT - FOODS TO AVOID DURING DETOX

This is a fun part-I discuss a few absolute do not eat foods. Reason being is that these foods will to cause you to keep suffering with your thyroid. Giving them up is a must and it only "hurts" at first then you transition off them and you feel too good to look back. Removing these offending foods is so you can both detox and heal. I will also give you some great tips that I use myself so that you can easily replace these foods.

How do you know when you are not well?

You begin to feel tired all the time. Some people have headaches, a racing heart, skin rashes, you begin to lose your hair, and you get cystic acne. Also, the Doctor confirms a diagnosis. All are what I call "lack of ease." If you are not at ease, pleasant, relaxed most of the time, joyful, able to sing on occasion, and breathe clean air, feel good, you begin to lack; eventually, it is patently obvious: dark circles under your eyes, weight issues/obese, your always in pain, swollen, you miss work and school, you have toxic disagreements with lots of people, you have anxiety and, depression, you must sit on the toilet and read because you're often constipated. These are what we pay attention to before we wait for the diagnosis.

Foods that are to be strictly avoided during your Detox:

1.     All wheat and gluten: rye, barley
2.     All dairy
3.     Factory Farmed animal products

When you detox you want to swerve on these three foods because:

1.    This food specifically causes anxiety and depression, bloating, gut damage, foul moods, digestion problems, and, congests your thyroid gland.

2.    Dairy is mucous and full of antibiotics, pesticides from bovine feed, vaccines and their chemicals, growth hormones, and, despair. Our feelings are the chemical messengers in  our blood and lymph fluids.

3.    Factory farmed animals similar to the dairy category are causing swelling, inflammation,   disease, bacteria like H Pylori Bacterium and the hormones are not healthy during our detox.

Wheat and gluten will make our scalp itch, tops of my feet will itch, my urine will become bubbly, and smell, and any of the three above will produce mucous that I can feel thinning and moving from my eyes, ears and nose, a clear mucous when I am in the shower. I can smell the stink immediately and begin to itch and feel uncomfortable. Additionally, I do not sleep as well and I begin to clear my throat! Mucous comes up and I get a slight feeling like a headache coming on near my temples.

Now, can you imagine how you may feel if you were not desensitized to eating these three things? And, if you had not grown up thinking they were just a normal everyday part of life? I mean just about everybody you meet is having pizza: wheat meat and cheese. Or, Mexican food, wheat, meat and cheese, and sandwiches, same thing, wheat, meat and cheese. Americans love their chicken! It's in everything, and these birds are so mutated in factory farms and full of a contagious bacteria. This means that once you are infected, you, are contagious too! You cannot just cook this bacteria out as with the other factors I list you consume them and, you become unwell.

I will cover a bit about each food you may not want to include during your detox and that will be entirely up to you. If you have a very minor thyroid problem and symptoms then you can remove the 3 foods and do the detox and if you have major symptoms and an autoimmune diagnosis like Hashimoto's Disease you may want a more thorough detox. I have had stellar results with people with autoimmune issues where they had very long term diagnosis and we worked together weekly in consults for about 6 months, so about 24 sessions in a package and reversed autoimmune with great clarity and tools up to 85%. Some clients got busy and indicated that they will be back after graduate programs or other times of their lives to go the full 100%.

We can sense when we are not entirely well and, when we do not have enough energy.  Calories (food), are energy, or, I should say *some* calories give the kind of energy that will fuel you and other calories will drain you. Your body will have to work especially hard to digest some of these foods, and, they are damaging to your gut. It is confusing to say the least, I realized that food, is business today and, in the last 100 years.

Two major industries: dairy and meat both used schools to establish programming. They supplied curriculum and coloring sheets for younger children that they would bring home and have their art at home that was colored by the children in school during the day and small milk cartons were brought in reinforcing that we need calcium from a cow. This could not be further from the truth, and, the sooner you realize this, the better! If you have any doubts, please, read The Calcium LIe2 by Dr. Robert Thompson. I highly encourage you to read his book, and learn about what calcium has been doing to you. It will amaze you and you will never want to use it again!

The Dairy and Meat Industries programmed young children for nearly 100 years with untruths that were a direct lie about calcium and protein. This programming is etched within the psyche of nearly everyone and you must look at the truth and then remove yourself from the propaganda created to form an allegiance with you and their products: living beings in cruel factory farm warehouses. This is, is part of waking up living fully, and detoxifying yourself from false information sold to you and your ancestors long ago.

Some people prefer to eat meat and I understand, especially if you are a hunter and you obtain your own wild food that is very different from commercial grocery store factory farmed animals full of chemicals, toxic heavy metals and hormones.

I have a story about a client of mine who experienced the pressure and conformity placed upon school children in American schools. She had an experience I want to share with you because when she shared it with me on day while in session with her it struck a chord-one I will never forget. She was a tender young girl in elementary school and a tray was brought in with very small containers, likely those little boxes that I can remember as well and everybody in the class was instructed to be sure to drink their milk! She drank her milk and then she had vomiting-not just vomiting but projectile vomiting. The next day she came to school again a little embarrassed that this had happened in front of her classmates and teacher. Again, the milk was brought into the classroom, under the assumption that it would "do a body good," and she refused the milk. The teacher told her she would drink the milk sternly! I realize many people are reading this right now with an expected response:

She was lactose intolerant. No, nobody digests bovine mammary fluid that has been pasteurized (heated to kill any nutrition in it) and homogenized (added cheap artificial vitamins that are toxic to it).

The young girl became upset and, she was told to get under the teacher's desk and into the garbage can and sit there; she was **humiliated**. She describes how she avoided class for some time and it changed her life in many ways.

I came to learn a lot about the family because I care about them deeply and I know they care about me too, we have built a trust. We trust our food industry, and all the other industries around us. Once you have completed this book, and you have detoxed yourself and healed your eyes may be greatly opened and you may begin a new chapter of your life.
**Humiliation, is the Mind Body trigger for thyroid imbalance.** Can you think of other instances of humiliation and lack of trust that could also be aspect of thyroid imbalance in our world?

### Breakfast, Lunch & Dinner

We have all absorbed many programs. As we progress into understanding and formulating our own personal detoxification and thyroid healing that we are putting together in our composition book and Food Diary, from time to time we must examine some of the programs and replace or update them.

People often assume that obese people eat too much and that they are overweight because of their sloppy habits. I believe that perhaps some people eat too much, but a large percentage of people who are obese or morbidly obese are lacking minerals and had a thyroid gland that went awry long ago as children and then, they were fed the foods on our list of 3 in large doses that caused them to dramatically balloon.

Many developed gastric and digestive "diseases" like Crohn's Disease, IBD, and had mysterious colon problems, yet they were no mystery to me. I saw the Mind Body, diet and lifestyle aspects of each and every one of them. And, you could tell for 3 decades now that a small minority comparatively believed that they are reversible, sadly. I have gained tremendous experience in seeing through the fraud, special language and the drugs now called "medications," most of the time.

Behind excess weight is always pounds of pain, and, programming. We are programmed in many ways we rarely give thought to but I believe are worthy of mention here: we are trained to **finish our plate**, even when we are full, this programming continues even today and has been in place for over 100 years to my knowledge. We are trained to feel as though we should have breakfast to get started on the day with energy when nothing could be further from the truth? I encourage my clients to start the day with fresh made juice if they can, or a blended drink and to begin as late as possible perhaps even 11 am. To drink warm tea, take your probiotic, allow your continued digestive and elimination channels to do the work they need to do, especially if you are sitting at a desk like I was for many years in a chair, compromising your digestion and elimination. Drink tea, then filtered water and then your juice or blended drink or smoothie. Get the fresh enzymes, minerals and key ingredients to make you sparkle!

70

One the upgrades to the standard breakfast program of starch, cheese, meat, or wheat is to prepare a freshly made large juice or blended drink, fruit salad or ACAI bowl which you can easily make in minutes.

If you do not have a juicer, let's put that in your composition book so you make a notation that this is a part of your detox plan and get this handled within the week.

You can get one at Walmart, or online through Craig's List, and many of my clients who were on a very tight budget placed an ad online and found one for $10 or found one at yard/garage sales locally. People get them, never use them and then put them in their basements or attic so just ask and you will have one!

**JUICE DIRECTION/RECIPE:** I like apple, **lemon or lime** and ginger: You need a juicer-centrifugal or masticating, depending upon your budget. First wash your produce, cut the **apple** in half or fourths to fit in your juicer **feed tube** and use the stem, the seeds (yes, I know they contain trace amounts of arsenic), and cut your citrus ends off the rough parts only and place it in the juicer feeding tube in halves or smaller if you need to, and take and slice the **ginger** piece of about 5-6" in length so it does not jam up your juicer cut it into about 8 slices and place them in and you will feel amazing, and, ginger as purported by a great many destroys cancer cells. Clear glass recycled juice jars, wide mouth mason jars (clear) work really well and keep you inspired by the beautiful colors you enjoy as your upgrade your mornings!

If you cannot get a juicer at this time, you can go to the dollar store and get a small citrus juicer that you can cut your lemon or lime and place the half of the citrus and squeeze and turn and place the juice of lemons, and limes in a larger container with filtered water and you can even add some pure maple syrup or a bit of coconut palm sugar, stevia or honey. You can also blend ginger and water with a sweetener as well too.

Number One reason people stop juicing? Cleaning the juicer! Just rinse it down if you are needing to get out the door early for work or school and clean it a bit better later on for 5 minutes or so. The benefits will quickly and direct outweigh cleaning the juicer.

**BLENDED DRINK DIRECTION/RECIPE:** I love cantaloupe and organic banana, it is simple, fast and delicious! It reminds me of an orange pop from long ago it is that sweet! It feels like a decadent treat too! Simply have your stock of cantaloupe for the upcoming week, buy 3-4 or more and place them in a sunny window to activate them unless they are really ripened and then you will want to place them in the refrigerator to preserve them from ripening further. Cut the cantaloupe in half with a large knife, then, gently scoop out the seeds (some people eat them for the

Omegas), so you preserve the sweetest part of the cantaloupe, it's good to place them in the Earth if you have a compose and give back, if not they go in the garbage. Cut the halves into chunks and then cut away the rind with your paring knife and discard it in the compost or the garbage. Add those chunks to your blender, and use a wooden spoon to help it get started as you turn it off briefly push down on the spoon to mush it just a bit and then it will blend up quite easily and nicely. Add 1-3 frozen organic bananas that you break into chunks (I freeze mine whole and peeled in freezer bags), and you have a thick, orange delicious, sweet blended drink. You can omit the bananas, you can add other superfoods like I do from time to time like **gelatinized maca root** to balance your hormones, or moringa powder, cacao powder, and vitamin C food based powder, ACAI powder all are delicious and you getting creative make this a lot of fun! I use blended drinks when I feel a bit done with cleaning my juicer for a bit and I need a break from the cleaning of it as well as summer time more often for cooler drinks.

**Lunch time** could be between 12-4 and, it could be your one large meal of the day. Your two hands placed or cupped together are your own **unique bowl** it is your portion of food for the day, except in today's world we eat for many reasons, and, often *empty calories* so we are left longing for more food. This is the time for me that I eat the food, and depending on the weather, the season, it will vary. If I am physically working a lot it may be something very easy on occasional bag of crimini mushrooms and a tub of roasted red pepper hummus to dip, or a spiral salad with organic hemp seed oil to pour atop and some good quality salt, it could be a leftover simple soup, or a wild rice dish with a fresh avocado to slice up. **Avocado is your fat source go to**! They are extremely healthy for your entire nervous system and they are easy to digest a lovely fruit!

Instead of **dinners** like we always had growing up on the Standard American Diet "SAD," the majority of us anyway, where we had a cold glass of cow milk, a small portion of veggies and a piece of meat, some brown potatoes mashed or scalloped in my home, we could upgrade and munch on some raw veggies and a simple dip like a Vegan Green Goddess dressing which is easily made: use your food processor 2 avocados, stick onion, olive oil, garlic, a bit of lemon juice, salt and pepper, and whatever else you wish to add, or, make your own simple hummus with those cooked garbanzo beans, in any flavor you wish: roasted red pepper, broccoli, garlic, I have even seen goji berry, cayenne and many other flavors. And, use up that zucchini into raw pies, salads, steamed veggies, or atop wild rice, in with some quinoa. The detox is to give you energy and give your thyroid gland a break from all the starch, mucous and toxins. I guarantee results if you follow along and it is quite easy to tell if people are not doing the detox. You have limitless choices and you can find even more at www.one-greenplanet.org so be sure to sign up for their email list and just pick recipes that are also gluten free.

You will be asked repeatedly, "where are you getting your protein?" And, "you look like you may be getting too thin?" And, "you won't be able to last eating like that!" I have heard them all and this protocol has saved my life more than once and the lives of many a client over decades.

I believe we have to rethink the programming and dominant language that causes expectation of Breakfast, Lunch and Dinner, and learn to feed our cells. Caloric restriction has been proven time and time again and, it's central clarity is that that we wear out our body from eating excessively. The only one to gain anything positive from that is the food industry! Wheat and other foods are actually designed to causing us to eat more food and more often; this, produces larger sales, larger waistlines and a more thyroid gland imbalance. Food coma happens by eating too much, especially when we are triggered: the night before returning to the job from hell, or the stress of the new daycare where you are forced to take your child, or any of the many stressors in our lives. We tend to eat heavily at night and then we do not sleep well, we wake tired and unrefreshed and moody, crunchy sleep eyes (mucous & starch), and, sit on the throne too long, wasting time, stinking up the bathroom, and, we take huge bowel movements because we overtaxed our gut, and elimination channels way too early in life pacifying ourselves with food; orally gratifying ourselves with food and "treating" ourselves with sweets for the missing sweetness in our lives-take this from an expert that learned from experience!

We are breaking our fast from our sleep where we were regenerating our cells, we want to feed our cells: sunlight, walking, filtered or distilled water, probiotic, fresh juice, food based vitamin C, 5HTP if necessary and a brief skin brushing and out the door we can go with our food in a recyclable tote or bag if we are working full time or students.

**THE ULTIMATE SANDWICH DIRECTIONS/RECIPE:** Make your wraps using **Nori** from the sea veggies section of the natural foods store, or, use a green leaf like collard green, Swiss chard, butter leaf lettuce, and add a simple dressing, or hummus, on the collard green with the hard spine removed with a knife and folded in half and soften the leaf with your hands a bit or a rolling pin. Place your sandwich contents, whatever that may be for you: fish, avocado, raw nuts like pine nuts, macadamia halves, sprouts, spinach, mushrooms, and you have a delicious wrap, and occasionally, I also use the brown rice spring roll wrappers as well, but more often I go for the green leaf, favoring the Swiss chard. I also bring seaweed to munch on for more bioavailable iodine and my absolute favorite is fresh sun dried Nori from The Seaweed Man online which comes in about one time per year! www.theseaweedman.com You can always make a plate for yourself as well using portobello mushroom/s and place your veggies or quinoa or black rice on top. Chop up some parsley or cilantro on top and always use some good quality Celtic or iodized sea salt to season which is great for your thyroid. What you do not want to use is sodium the white salt devoid of nutrients.

### Salt

There is a lot of misinformation floating around about salt. I like salt and it adds flavor to a lot of my foods and, I also went long years without adding any kind of salt because of being on a very careful and strict Ital diet. The Ital diet comes from Jamaica and involves eating foods from the Earth without the use of salt. In part, because Haile Selassie warned the African people about the use of salt in the form of sodium which is most commonly found today in restaurants and the salt packets people receive in drive up fast food restaurants. Many food items were salted for preservation and they caused health problems, unlike iodized salts. Sodium is detrimental and salt with iodine is beneficial. Oftentimes depending on the severity to detox, I will have a client drink a quart of water with a 1/4 to 1/2 teaspoon of good quality iodized Celtic or Redmond sea salt as often as three times per day. I also absolutely enjoy the **sulfur rich black salt** (Kala Namak), which I use liberally even though it felt really odd for me at first, and it may for you too to use salt when I have avoided it so much for so many years. Once I was detoxed and did not have as much swelling salt was very healing and restorative. If you remember way back, our parents had us gargle with salt water to cure our problems with our gums and teeth and we often use salt water for balancing.

Be sure to enjoy your salt!

### Wheat & Gluten

You have to give this up! And, it sounds odd like it would not make that much of a difference but it does, a huge difference and you will feel it. You know all those people, maybe you? Who pick at their face, their scalp, have dandruff, itch all the time, have ruddy skin, lots of stomach problems, yep, it's the wheat and gluten!

It's everywhere and seems pretty weird that with a bestselling book out there; hoping people actually read it? That we do not have more changes than I see currently? A few places offer gluten free and dairy free foods, obviously, we are not sending a loud enough message as to what we, the consumer want.

When I first learned the significance of our food industry upon our body, mind and spirit I felt certain that we would all shift gears into eating real food, and, with a youthful exuberance in my 20s, I bought and passed around the video on VCR then, called Diet for A New America.

There was a natural foods store, Staff of Life in Santa Cruz, CA which had a small area with a few tables, one of the tables was a long rectangle where I often came and ordered through the small kitchen window one of several choices: brown rice, cashew gravy and steamed veggies. We had a community table where we could eat together with whomever was at the store cafe. There was Gomasio which is a blend that I later learned about in Ayurvedic training with Cynthia Copple at White Lotus, as well as large container of nutritional yeast flakes that we could liberally put on our rice giving it a cheesy flavor. Lots of people that were far from the mainstream and many dreadlocks came to eat there healthfully. Plant based ways with low grain consumption or, no grain consumption are lower in plaque in our arteries, our brain, our hearts, our bowel and cutting out wheat and gluten we have far less congestion in the body that directly affects our thyroid gland.

When I think about where I want to go eat, Dharma's in Capitola does it for me, in the Midwest, there is nothing like it! Ecopolitan which was 100% raw, was a favorite in Minneapolis it was absolutely amazing and I went on a retreat with the owner last year, however, it's now closed sadly. You may find after your detox and healing that you open a pop up restaurant like Facebook friend NURAH Stanley in Michigan, which is vegan and entirely "electric," following the good works of Dr. Sebi.

Today, if drive across country as I have done so many times, between California and Minnesota you see a Nation replete with the same "chains." I use that word sound intentionally, because they will chain you, the burgers, 'fries' GMO potatoes, dairy products: milkshakes, coffee drinks, sour cream, potatoes, ranch dressing packets and, the other toxic offerings are precisely the reason why you have migraines, headaches, skin rashes, thyroid problems, and, the persistent mornings feeling like 'crap.' For many people they awaken to feelings of near suicidal thoughts, deep depression and compound that with daily wheat use (remember, it's a drug), and mornings are not as pleasant as they could be. You are reading along with me and so I can see that you will bring about change and heal yourself!

Wheat is a culprit that is a major piece of thyroid imbalance and anxiety, depression and suicides. We feed wheat to the poor like nobody's business. Wheat, is not food. The birthday cake, can easily be replaced with other options using almond or coconut flour. I was just relating with my cousin this morning about how to make her rhubarb bars without using wheat flour. Why would we not get our children off of government surplus food like wheat? When you take children off wheat, dairy and factory farmed animal products, you get an increase in attention, comprehension, alertness, and the decreases impulsivity, inattention, fidgeting and much more! Imagine our children eating real food! But then they wouldn't be medicated as often?

First, begin to notice where wheat is, what products have it, and, then, avoid wheat and gluten until you can omit it entirely with your willpower! Anybody with thyroid concerns simply must abandon wheat to avoid the congestion-the way **it irritates the throat, esophagus, and the gut.** **BUT I WAS CHECKED AND I DO NOT HAVE CELIAC?** This can be confusing for people because they may think that they have already ruled out Celiac or gluten intolerance? Many, had a procedure done-where a doctor examines your inner gut in a procedure often done with a colonoscopy called an endoscopy. They use a type of a camera that goes down into the gut and look for irritation consistent with dermatitis or lymphoma of the gut and if they do not see it then you can still go eat the wheat and gluten and come back again.

Many people eat wheat and gluten, every single day: muffins, pancakes, sandwiches, tortillas, burritos, toast, stuffing, and more! Their doctors told them they were not gluten intolerant or "Celiac".

Over many years now, I find that every single person who gives up wheat recovers quickly and never looks back, it's getting off this drug which is on every corner that is the hard part! Let me explain: you walk down the street and the sandwich shop has it, the Mexican restaurant has it on the tortillas, the doughnut shop, the bread bakery, just about everywhere, including your friend who has pasta on the menu tonight for dinner! One way to get off this killer and I did choose my words very carefully, is to remember: Pasta is paste! It clogs you and causes you a lot of problems including indigestion, colon problems, gut problems, gas, and stomach distention, and, it's often a part of those "bowling ball" bellies that we see on so many men today. Wheat is additionally, causing a lot of our obesity epidemic and you see the effects of wheat on our children today with those off color, white, crusty patches or, "wheat patches" on their facial skin and body, Dermatitis you just need to start focusing in on how bad it truly is, maybe read The Wheat Belly book because eating wheat will even cause Dermatitis Lymphoma that occurs in the gut and, produces bleeding ulcers.

In the book, The Wheat Belly and so many others, it is worthy of mention that people who have long suffered with migraines, headaches, and all sorts of problems, cleared themselves from these problems in one week.

I think I honestly have the most stubborn family members on the planet. Close family members have Thyroid Cancer, including removal of the entire gland, Generalized Anxiety Disorder which is the "check engine light," that precedes a thyroid diagnosis.

Now, if the wheat was not bad enough, lurking even further in the **food-to-hospital pipeline.** Nearly all products sold as food, made from flour today are brominated and that, is a halogen which is highly disruptive to our thyroid gland. Add insult to injury right? Now, let's imagine for a moment. Folks go into the convenience store and grab an egg sandwich under the heat lamp, and, a Mt. Dew or energy drink to get their day going. However, the wheat, bromine in the sandwich, the "cheese food," on the egg sandwich, the scrambled egg "protein" that is rancid and the brominated drink is a big hazard to the thyroid gland. What are we doing to stop this madness? We could just stop purchasing these things and steering people out of this trickery-we could begin to educate if our students were learning how to grow food, feed themselves and conserve, become sustainable and educated in how to stay out of debt and live with more conscious movement: building their own shelters, and not just going into academic/student debt right out of the proverbial adult "gate," into the world. If we educate them to stay away from food drugs that kill them slowly we all win. More productive, less suicidal, mood disordered, cancer, autoimmune, violent people.

What about social eating? How do we go out to eat? I feel rude at other people's homes that invite us over to eat with them and prepare lovely meals? Well, fortunately, now that its "official" and you can comfortably say, I cannot eat wheat, to which you get a predictable response, "Oh, you have allergies? Or, are you "Celiac?" you have allergies to wheat?"

And, I say, "I just don't eat wheat, it's dangerous." And, people may look at you depending upon your answer and wonder what you mean, and you can share with them that there are entire courses on why you should avoid wheat and gluten which means:

Wheat, Rye, and Barley. Barley! One of my favorite soups to make, ugh, but, I found so many great substitutes that again, I'm not going to leave you in the lurches of wondering what on earth you are going to do to have some semblance of "normal," life!

Be sure to avoid using the "fake meats," that are made with seitan, which is wheat and gluten as you can utilize the jackfruit, as well as other healthier options. Years ago when I began taking vegan cooking classes in 1982 at The Bread of Life in Campbell, CA, the ladies, many of which had goat farms taught us how to make nut loaf, black bean burgers, and there are other ways including using garbanzo, otherwise called "chickpea" patties, burgers, strips. People transitioning off of eating animals can begin to make recipes using beans, wild rice, sweet potatoes and other foods even without a recipe. I found it quite easy to get comfortable with using other sources like those easily found in natural foods stores.

First, I get a general gluten free flour to keep on hand, I like Bob's Red Mill stuff a lot but I avoid the mixes now that have very high starch. If you look at the ingredients and you see potato starch and tapioca starch in the top 5, I tend to go with almond flour or coconut flour whenever I can and my favorite for savory recipes is Bob's Redmill Garbanzo Bean Flour and, it's typically only $2.99 per bag. I make vegan omelets and a tortilla type of pancake for a wrap or just to enjoy with a fresh guacamole and/or cilantro. It could not be easier! I get out a mixing bowl, add in my spices, some filtered water, some aluminum free baking powder and whip it up let it sit for about 15 minutes with a clean dish towel over the top and then lightly do them on a flat grill with very importantly: grape seed oil is the secret!

I also use teff flour for pancakes and teff for hot cereal so you do have choices to have something that feels familiar! For soups, use garbanzo beans, wild rice, veggies and your juicing pulp which you can blend or use your food processor and then place in ice cube trays and freeze up in a freezer bag for later use for soups to maximize your investments in food and make a healthy broth.

## Soy

Soy is most often genetically modified (GMO), and, it is high on the list of goitrogenic foods which means that it irritates the thyroid gland. There is a lot of people checking into this but, I would avoid it as a mainstay for sure. I use a stash in a warm tea if there is no other option very infrequently, and, I also rarely enjoy some edamame at Japanese restaurants or out and about because it is pretty few and far between that I partake of soy. At one time, in the 1980s I was consuming a lot of soy in the form of daily soy milk, tofu and tempeh and was informed that in addition to my hormonal imbalances that were forming it was not the best idea to consume soy as heavily as I once was so I took a long break from it and replaced it with other choices. Every great once in a while I will eat a bit of tofu for memory sake but it's not a good investment.

Soy milk which is most often the alternative "creamer" for our coffee, tea, at many delis, soy burgers, and the soy sauce for Chinese food which contains simple sodium all have replacements. Other nut milks are an option and one of my favorite is pumpkin seed milk, there are creamers available now that are made from coconut, as well as hundreds of ways to make "burgers" using beans, nuts, and, tamari instead of soy sauce.

## Corn

I love corn, I truly do! I love polenta, corn on the cob, and cornbread for sure, however, it is pretty rare that I enjoy corn today largely because of how it has been changed and how my digestion will 'interpret' this non food when it goes down the hatch, affecting my esophagus and the sphincter which is easily damaged for a great many people who in America especially today, "overfeed." Corn is delicious and a staple grain found in most of our cereals, many of our products and it is part of our ritual, celebrations, and family traditions to have cornbread, corn on the cob with summer BBQs. What do we do if we get rid of corn?

I related above that I use chickpea flour and chickpeas in general, in fact soaking them you can sprout them and eat them that way if your digestion is pretty sturdy, you can cook them up and use the water "Aquafaba" as your new binder in your recipes like an egg would be

**Dairy**

Look at convenience stores and standard grocery stores and most people leaving have a gallon or more of milk. Milk has two meanings: it the mammary gland fluid rich in fat and protein as well as it means to exploit or defraud (someone). Milk is now a universal term used to refer to one fluid: bovine. According to www.organicconsumers.org

Over the last 50 years, the way food animals are raised and fed has changed dramatically surprised to find that most of the food animals in the United States are no longer raised on farms at all. Instead they come from crowded animal factories, also known as large confined animal feeding operations (CAFOs).

Just like other factories, animal factories are constantly searching for ways to shave their costs. To save money, they've redefined what constitutes animal feed, with little consideration of what is best for the animals or for human health. As a result, many of the ingredients used in feed these days are not the kind of food the animals are designed by nature to eat.

Just take a look at what's being fed to the animals you eat.

Same Species Meat
Diseased Animals
Feathers, Hair, Skin, Hooves, and Blood
Manure and Other Animal Waste
Plastics
Drugs and Chemicals
Unhealthy Amounts of Grains

Are these ingredients legal? Unfortunately, yes. Nevertheless, some raise human health concerns. Others just indicate the low standards for animal feeds. But all are symptoms of a system that has lost sight of the appropriate way to raise food animals.

Multiple generations carry a program. The program repeats itself over and over, unless and until someone takes a moment to observe beyond the rote way of doing what we do every day. We call it introspection because you come inside your own self and you think about dairy for a moment, and how programmed you are, or, were and how the appeal to group mentality and persuasion is everywhere, like a beacon. In every store you find cow milk, yogurt, cottage cheese, a variety of cheeses, sour cream, ice cream, hot chocolate mixes, and more. Not only is it overwhelming for the person considering the change to embrace that this product sold by stores, having come from the feedlots or factory farms is entirely toxic, pasteurized, and most often in toxic containers, but it also congests and congeals you due to the 50 years or more, of indiscriminate treatment of these animals. These animals are suffering from the same thing humans are: encephalopathy which means in short, swollen brains.

Mucous is a good thing right? Yet out of your nose, ears, pores and your anus is not so great and we can see that when we shower, sauna and as well as when you are "sick."

Cheese is seriously like crack to try to give up, it is so addicting and, it is made using casein most of the time which is an excitotoxin and overworks your neurons in your brain and then leaves your exhausted and depleted. But just as I will continue to do, you can do an upgrade and make delicious plant and nut based cheeses as there are so many delicious recipes that are 4-5 ingredients online, especially at a website I enjoy so much! www.one-greenplanet.org, if you go and subscribe you will get emailed great articles, easy often vegan and gluten free recipes and pictures to get you started with a fresh supply of healthful ideas. And, occasionally when I am not making a raw cashew "cheese," I will occasionally use nutritional yeast but, sparingly like a small dusting on a dish for a slight cheese look and taste. You can find that as nutritional yeast flakes (I like the large vs. the small flakes) in the bins at the natural foods stores.

### Factory Farmed Meat & Nitrates

Any of the products like jerky, lunch meats, hot dogs, brats, and many other injected meats like hams, sausages you must look for "nitrate free," on the label if you eat animal products otherwise this makes everything swell with inflammation in the body and that is not good for your thyroid as well.

Dogs as well, please consider that often the nitrates in the snacks we give them in the form of the inexpensive beef sticks found at the counter of convenience stores not only have nitrates but also the notorious red food dye that I found to be the antagonist for seizures for dogs quite often. Look for nitrate free products which are found more often now, even in convenience stores.

### Eggs

The Standard American Diet typically consisted of a classic menu that most people had for meals and eggs were on most people's plates for breakfast, especially on the weekends. People enjoy their food, I know I do, and we have become accustomed to certain expressions have become familiar expressions like: "eggs sunny side up," "scrambled." Eggs are used for cake recipes for birthdays, we poached them, had Eggs Benedict, Eggs Florentine and with all manner of sauces like hollandaise and in gourmet brunch locations, however, for me, and many of my clients the histamine of eggs and the toxicity of the factory farming industry has us making the choice to abandon eggs. I miss the taste, but not the many deciding factors for me which caused me to quit consuming them, except for the dogs in their raw state.

People who have so many allergies, asthma, sinusitis, lung issues, skin rashes and more, need to detox and then make a decision for yourself, once you are detoxed a good bit you may find that you do just fine and you buy your eggs somewhere like a local farm or outside of the factory farms so that you are getting a better egg than from distressed beings fed commercial feed and boxed up without sunlight, possibly fed antibiotics in large doses and so forth. You may return to eggs, you can decide after you detox. Many people dissuade about breaking the yoke as Dr. Thompson claims that it makes for a rancid protein and you can find out more about that in his book, The Calcium Lie 2.

### Coffee & Barista Drinks Containing Syrups

For as much as like being able to get a nice hot beverage on a cold day and just get out among people and enjoy the day, I have to find a place that offers a drink that I will not pay the price for consuming later! What I mean is that most of the drinks today are made using syrup pumps that contain numerous ingredients that inflame the body, sadly again.

Whether you go to Starbucks, Caribou, or any of the many coffee, and tea houses, a great majority of them do not make real products any longer. They offer just about all wheat donuts, bagels, pastries, and sliced beautiful loaves of banana, pumpkin, and other breads, cake pops, and croissant type sandwiches, and all of these coffee establishments carry the same processed foods that are high in sugar, wheat and likely brominated flour. The syrups are a problem as they full of sugar and artificial colors which typically cause me to heat up soon after consuming the fake flavors that they add to lattes, mochas, pumpkin flavored drinks, and even chai today is just a horrid mix of artificial syrup pumped into a fluid and packaged up as the real deal. It makes you sweat and is not healthy at all! It is a whole lot better to make up your own chai, your own herbal tea in a mason jar or make up some Dandy Blend which is dandelion leaves which is a great liver tonic and easy to find online, or, Teeccino which I have used in years past and really liked a lot!

Coffee is very acidic and I notice that while I absolutely love the taste and the occasional use to  get driving a bit longer on the road, or finish a project, with full knowledge that I'm using a drug (caffeine), I want to avoid it. It produces lumps and I notice that when I drink it I feel breast tenderness and clients have reported the same thing. Often people are desensitized by way of consuming it daily and so they are not as in tune with what they feel from regular consumption. Coffee is known to be an antagonist for our thyroid gland and you have other options to find something a bit more healthy.

### Processed Foods

You know, once you get in the habit of eating well, what I call a "food rhythm," and you get your shopping done on the weekend, placing your fresh fruit and vegetables out where you see and use them and you budget your meals. You develop a habit of using all that you purchase, and not wasting, as well as making that fresh food every single day. It's far easier to get into the habit of cutting up a cantaloupe in the morning, add a handful of spinach, or a pineapple and some swiss chard and getting it blended and into a large recycled glass jar that holds you and nicely takes care of the morning if you are headed out to work or school and then by lunch time you have a great salad packed up for yourself or other options like spiral sliced salad with a lovely dressing and a nice high fat avocado chopped up with a handful of raw sunflower seeds or, Brazil nuts to get our selenium levels up which aids our thyroid gland: ideally, 3-6 raw brazil nuts per week so just buying a super small fresh refrigerated baggy of brazil nuts will help you get more bioavailable vitamins to help you and your brain too!

### Food Additives:

Colorants, especially ones that come from insects like the red food dye, the artificial flavors and the other additives to make you want to come running back for more, do more than make you feel for food when you are not hungry-they damage your gut and your thyroid gland. And, many ingredients

### Starch Stiff

Ever wonder why some people really crack and creak when they get up in the morning: everything from their toes to their joints in their knees, and all over? I mean, you can hear and see what starch stiff is with many people on the massage table just working on stiff feet, lifting their arms, their shoulder joints will all be stiff and click loudly into place just putting their arm back down on the table? This is because they are starch stiff! And, in homes where people eat white or brown rice with every meal, or, brown potatoes ,pasta and dairy many times per week, people build up a lot of cooked starch in their entire body-all over!

If you want to get rid of this you will have to intentionally lay off the starch until you detox it out and then, slowly integrate baked sweet potatoes—occasionally. Probably not the best idea to rely too heavily on starch rich meals if you want to wake up in the morning and not be as stiff, nor have the swelling in your joints.

What can you do to replace all the starch that most of us eat as winter comes around? It is not easy to drive by the delicious Chinese restaurant or the amazing Indian buffet for me, it's very difficult to turn down some of my favorite foods like Naan which is a bread that you dip your chickpea dishes, veggies, coconut curries and veggie stews! During the colder months especially, we want something warm and nourishing but also something that feels grounding, that is a heavier food for the colder weather. Foods that are high starch, like rice or brown potatoes are delicious and affordable, and this is where I turn to wild rice, which is not a rice at all and digests really well as well as has many nutrients and less starch, higher in protein and lower in carbohydrates. I occasionally eat the blue or purple potatoes that re called fingerlings.

We have a dish up this way that many people crave which I had never heard of called "Tater Tot Hotdish." If you want to assault your thyroid gland in one meal this would be the way to do it! Canned soups are deadly, canned foods are completely dead and so you are eating some calories but no nutrients. Perhaps for a survival event, but not a daily way of life. This is not an insult this is to help you and not mince words about it. Boxed, bagged and canned will not heal you; they will fill your gut, however, they will not provide you with enzymes, minerals and they may even harm your thyroid due to the toxic layer around the tin or can to prevent rust and mold for lots of storage time, including riding on hot trucks being shipped to your store for sale. Cheese, ground cow, and processed brown potatoes, together with cans of soup would sicken people and later, they would tell you they have allergies, the flu or a cold and, that, is the truth!

A raw diet which reduces inflammation more quickly, and is often a bit more low calorie, high enzyme diet from a clean food source without pesticides and sprays will heal people. You do not have to stay on it for all of your life, but you can use it to heal yourself on a temporary basis and then just make sure you eat clean, meaning many people hunt like my family members because they want meat and many people make cheeses from alternate sources: I do, that are plant based for my gluten free lasagna that I love to enjoy, and so this is not about converting you into something that is too hard to do, it is about giving you the tools that actually work to heal your thyroid right now over a relatively short period so you can likely avoid taking medications and then notice the signs that show up that I have presented like you should become your own physician first: notice your tongue periodically during the week, notice your urine color and your bowel movements are they everyday? Are they pebbles, logs, what color are they? Notice the skin on your arms do you have spots, hyper pigmentation, do you sweat, do you sweat too much? This becomes as automatic for me as I do not "spend" my quality time in front of a TV, I gave it up in 1985 as it was suggested to me that I would enhance the quality of my life, and, it has, significantly! I highly recommend it, you will hear the news from people trust me. But you will have the time, people say they do not have to skin brush for a minute, make your juice or blended drink and walk just replacing the glazing over most people do in front of a radiation box dispelling poor role models, drugs, and, negativity most of the time.

### Sea Veggies & Seaweed

Over half the people I have consulted with over the decades have tried Japanese food, or had some form of sushi, and many have now tried seaweed salad, or the rolls many people make with a variety of ingredients using Nori, or simple seaweed salads using wakame, some toasted sesame oil, sesame seeds, thin sliced carrots, but there are so many varieties of seaweeds that are not just food as medicine but they make common sense as it relates to our sustainability-they heal your thyroid in many ways. You see, both of your thyroid hormones that are known as "T3," and "T4," are made up of 3 and 4 iodine parts respectively. You need and want iodine and it is a huge reason why so many people are having thyroid issues today, but not just thyroid; issues originating from thyroid that are now a result of thyroid imbalance and the cysts made by the body protectively to prepare from the onslaught of halides: chlorine, bromine and fluoride that are used far too much in the world today, they compete for iodine and so leave your thyroid and thyroid hormones without what it needs!

Eat your seaweed and develop a habit of trying a new type and way to prepare it so that you get familiar with it and comfortable knowing what to do with it. I began by making simple soups! Filtered water, cut up some kelp with kitchen scissors, added a handful of DULSE, added some iodized sea salt, a few spices like onion powder, garlic powder, some green onions, carrots, broccoli, mushrooms and I have a soup in no time flat!

Talk about the perfect to go food to carry in your purse! sea veggies, like nori, and seaweed like pulse are super easy to carry them with you, use them, get used to them and how they impart what we began calling food as medicine a long while ago, "bioavailable," which is another way for saying they get what you need, in this case, Iodine and trace minerals into your body for your use instead of taking everything by capsule, pill, tincture or supplement of some way or form. Yes, you can eat sea veggies and seaweed, and, they are super delicious; one of my personal favorites is the sun dried Atlantic Nori from The Seaweed Man in Maine. It looks a lot like something you are already familiar with: Beef Jerky and it is salty, chewable, and you can take it with you on hikes, so that you eat your medicine. The first time I ate a piece I could not believe how much I instinctively loved it, craved it, and feel that I needed it. What is difficult for most people who have this the first time is that it is different, it requires adapting. A pair of kitchen scissors and you could cut it up and place it on a wet salad where it would soften a bit, if you are not fond of eating it like jerky. You could cut it up a bit and place it in soups.

Eating the real Nori unlike what we have experienced at Japanese restaurants is delicious! It is looks like a piece of beef jerky and is really tasty! I crave it. The stuff that we have our sushi on and buy at natural food stores and Asian groceries, is a processed food that is pressed flat. It is not available all year round, but if you are lucky you can order it during the summer and then cherish it as I do!

There is always a little bit of a learning curve to produce change. Seaweeds will really bring you value in terms of their mineral content. One of the reasons that Japanese women experience far less incidence of breast cancers and had far less obesity, is due to their iodine consumption. People are unfamiliar with the texture of seaweeds, even if they like the salty nature of this food, we can learn to find either a soup, salad, sushi roll or something that we can find agreeable to get used to bringing seaweed into our diet.

We get iodine, and trace minerals from many seaweeds; iodine is crucial for detoxing your body, helping remove all those cysts, and, gain better thyroid function. There is iodine available in good quality sea veggies and seaweeds. And, you can take some of them on the go and easily integrate them into your day in many ways. Some of my favorite are: broth, soups, as stock for making wild rice, and, I cook some of them and chop them up and place them into spiral salads. Not only do they add the quality of aesthetics and a beautiful green color to the plate or bowl, but they are powerful detoxifiers! Iodine is crucial to detoxifying your internal organs!

Kelp is high in iodine and it matters which area you obtain it from, as I learned from The Seaweed Man, Larch, that kelp from the pacific coast is somewhat different in iodine content than from the Atlantic coast-as compared to Iceland, the iodine is a bit too high. Larch harvests his own seaweed, sun dries it and also, has a great cookbook. I have thoroughly enjoyed his quality products which are for sale on his website. He and his partner Nina have beautiful photography of their seaweed there and you get a feel for partaking in their lifestyle, as you view their pictures and videos. People can connect with them and do an apprenticeship

Kelp can be integrated into your diet on a daily basis, or, if you're like me, you will want to vary the types you consume as I share in this section. Alaria, Digitata Kelp is more commonly called "Kombu" in the natural foods stores but as Larch related with me, it is often bleached and takes from the quality of the seaweed. Dulse is one of my absolute favorites, I eat it like sea veggie jerky, it is easy to take along with you like jerky, dry, and easy to cut with kitchen shears and place into your salads, for high mineral content, as well as pack in my snack skins bags and keep in my purse or backpack in the event I find myself hungry, I always have something to munch on. It adds color to my food, salads, and, also adds that salty flavor I long for when I often forego dressings on a salad.

One thing I love about seaweeds is that it literally takes me 10 minutes when home on a break from work to add seaweeds like dulse and kelp to a pan of filtered water and a pinch of sea salt and I have a lovely broth in 10 minutes or I can simmer it on the stove when at home and enjoy the aromatherapy of a healthy broth as I add in carrots, stick onions, or whatever else I have to add to my pot of soup. People ask me all the time how to make a soup. I add a handful of kelp and a handful of dulse and my filtered water, a pinch of salt and then chop the veggies and Viola! It's soup!

The Seaweed Man also has a Soup Mix that is a convenient chopped blend of 50% Digitata Kelp, 25% Alaria and 25% Kelp which is super handy to have in a glass mason jar and be able to make a quick broth or soup.

Bladderwrack which is an excellent tonic for hypothyroid. They also sell a form of seaweed called rock weed which is used for fertilizer or animal supplementation that many places also sell as Irish moss.

Irish moss and Nori are often sold during the summer only as available.

My experience most of my life with seaweed was pretty minimal. I had commercially prepared Nori with sushi and vegetarian sushi rolls and I had drinks made with Irish moss by a few Jamaican folks and had heard that the "Moss" really is a tonic for men for their backbone and sexual stamina. I enjoyed the coconut milk variety with cinnamon and spices as well as the "herbal" which also contained cannabis back in the day in the early 1990s, however, I began to make them myself and also learn a lot more about this tonic even before I realized what it was doing for my thyroid gland.

Moss is so easy to use: You can find it online sold by TerraSoul and other places, including purple moss found in Jamaica. Look for nutrient rich sources, that are hand picked and sun dried. First, take out a handful and place it in a ceramic or glass bowl to soak in some filtered or distilled water. It is easily soaked for hours, or, overnight in order to remove any sand. Next, strained off the water and rise it well, and place it into a pan with clean filtered or distilled water and then cooked, (on medium for perhaps 20 minutes or so). Cooking is brief and just enough to remove the nutrients and the gel from the Moss so that it has the nutrients and thickening that Moss is so famous for! Last, remove the moss and either cook it again to make the gel, or throw it away or compost it. The liquid when cooled in the refrigerator will become a gel. That gel is what we add to the smoothies, and, I have even added it to make my raw pies including a cooked rhubarb pie with a raw crust made this summer. While you will have to experiment with it a bit you can increase the mineral content of your foods, again, making your food medicine. The gel is a great thickener for many recipes, both raw and cooked, savory as well as sweet recipes go well with Moss.

I absolutely love sea veggies and seaweeds. I encourage you to buy a family pack and perhaps a pound of dulse that is good quality and just get started incorporating them into your daily diet. In this way, you will get magnesium, iodine, and other trace minerals from your food in bioavailable ways that will detox and benefit you. Most people have no idea about how to integrate these types of foods into their diet, but now, you do!

Experiment with new ideas and recipes on your own as well! Adding color, minerals and great texture. If you are uncomfortable with the kelp, know that I was at first too. I took my time to use what I had and got out a cutting board (bamboo) and a good sharp sturdy knife and I chopped the kelp into smaller, finer pieces and begin to use it on top of a potato, in a salad, soup, spiral salad, seaweed salad with wakame which is one of my favorite seaweeds in terms of taste. I buy the wakame at the natural foods store and soak it briefly and then pull it out with a fork and add some toasted sesame seed oil and a bit of sliced avocado, fresh tomato, or whatever else I have and really enjoy it.

Detoxing and food are pretty simple. We want to avoid the commercial, super processed foods, wheat, the GMO foods like corn and soy, and the factory farmed animal products. For sure we want to avoid dairy, and, because it is so congesting and congealing for our throat and thyroid gland, for our health entirely! But also because using dairy products throws off our mineral balance by offsetting the body with calcium that is not useful to the body, and is actually harmful: it produces bone spurs and more! We want to rethink eating 3 big meals per day and the whole concept of Breakfast, Lunch and Dinner and move into fewer calories. In order to detox and heal our thyroid it is highly beneficial to start your day with a freshly prepared juice or blended drink to gain fresh nutrients, enzymes and minerals and to incorporate a food based Vitamin C powder as one of our supplements to detox and heal the body tissues and cells.

Also to regenerate our glands we want to get daily fresh vegetables which are grounding and recharging as well as balancing, and we can easily and quickly make salads with a spiral slicer using squash, sweet potato, onion, beets and more! Fresh salads with Swiss chard, and using raw vegetables with easy to make dips including avocado based Green Goddess or a hummus to use as a dip or dressing. Using raw nuts and seeds to make our milk, cheeses, as well as supplement for protein on a salad is ideal and a better choice than animal products during our detox for our thyroid and non-factory farmed meat and fish can be added back to the diet after your detox and achieving your goals and stabilize the body. Learn to vary the foods, fresh, local and in season is best for sustainability. Use sea weeds, sea veggies, broths, soups, smoothies, and remove wheat from the diet, replacing it with coconut flour, almond meal or flour, and garbanzo bean flours to transition out of a highly destructive food that is found almost everywhere and causes many of our health problems including Diabetes and other issues to the body.

# CHAPTER NINE - DETOX IS A LIFESTYLE

Sometimes our lifestyle habits are just a part of what we do everyday and we do not always think about many of our daily habits. I will cover some things that you will benefit from knowing so that you can further detox and heal your thyroid.

Detoxification tips relative to our lifestyle is equally important to our thyroid success and I will cover a great many that involve everyday habits for many people that I know you will benefit from and more quickly recover thyroid health and balance the result of becoming aware and implementing into your everyday life.

You have got to detox to be able to clear these halogens out of your tissues, and your thyroid gland that are blocking your ability to heal. Detox so your thyroid gland can receive and use the iodine. Remove harmful cookware like teflon, aluminum pots and pans and get rid of them.

Most chewing gums, lubricants, adhesives, preservatives used for shrimp and many seafoods, many shampoos, plastics, sleepwear for children, are all a part of our lifestyle today that is toxic. It is not a matter that people can't stop using them, it is that they won't stop using them.

### Aspirin & Pain Relievers

If you detox your cells, bones, organs, tissues, blood, and release mucous from your body, antagonists, and congestion you feel as though you have a new lease on life! I have learned a lot about detoxification in the last three plus decades and it has saved my life. I observed what detoxification did for my clients, and, how quickly they were able to heal. Through consults many were entirely able to reverse autoimmune. Most of our Elders are being instructed to take either a "blood pressure medication," "blood thinner," or Aspirin. Often, the need for any of these drugs is eliminated with detoxification and healing. I do not trust these drugs for long term use, and, I also understand where they seem to make sense for most people who will continue to eat wheat, consume dairy, and eat factory farmed animals. People are obese, swollen, inflamed and congested and often they do not know that they are creating this problem—no matter what you say, some will not even listen to reason? Aspirin was studied and has been shown to reduce thyroid hormone levels.

Why not thin down your body by doing do the detox and get off the foods I guide you to avoid? I would love to see the many places that care for people begin to offer real and simply prepared foods, as many elders who are not in charge of their own food, and people who live in assisted living, geriatric centers, as well as children in daycare, preschools, juvenile centers, hospitals, and more, eat the foods I specifically warn you against! Then, they "medicate" the various conditions caused by the food products.

Over the counter NSAIDs are bad news. They destroy your gut and they are a bandage to be used in a rare instance when there is no other option, yet today, we each have a bottle and take them far too often.

**Additionally drugs used for depression like Prozac contain fluoride! Fluoride blocks iodine from getting into the cells.**

### The Shower

Most people shower every single day in city municipal water that is treated with chlorine and often additionally has an additional halide: fluoride. Fortunately, we can install a shower filter, but most of them do not filter out fluoride. You are fortunate if you live in the country and have well water without the added chlorine and many contaminants. To shower or not to shower? If you ask most people they are not going to give up their shower.

The shower is an important aspect that we must cover with regard to examining our lifestyle aspects of detoxification because, if we shower every day or even multiple times per day not only does this dry out our skin's "mantle," but if we are showering under City water we are exposing ourselves to yet more halogens. City water systems are rife with lead, manganese like reported in our little city just last year (2016).

What can we do? We have other options: we can sponge bathe, which is what people often did years ago, where they use a wash cloth, wash the face, the underarms and the private areas. If you have never tried this, I encourage you to try it on a weekend, just give your skin a rest from the chlorine that dries it out, especially in the winter when we dry out a bit more from heaters going inside our homes, schools and office.

When we eat "clean" there is not the rancid body odor that accompanies eating a toxic diet with heavy processed foods, lots of coffee, soft drinks, items baked in aluminum foil which increase the toxicity, and factory farmed meats. A more plant-based diet which is so very simple to do and which reduces your calories is ideal- and optimizes your ability to sponge bathe as a viable option as opposed to showering all the time.

The shower can be used less frequently, at first, you can shower every other day as many people do.

## The Pits

If you are a guy, well, you're expected to have pit hair! But a woman on the other hand, well, there are some expectations that are cultural and familiar but they are always healthiest. We have armpit hair for a reason: we have about 20 lymph nodes under our arms and your armpit is actually an extension of your microbiome.

You can forego the underarm shaving once you are not stinking as much and opt for trimming the hair under your arms with scissors. You can keep them nice and trim but still have some of the hair. People again, are creatures of habit and, over the many years I have come to know the reaction of most people to this: yuck, and, gross! The further we move away from our Nature, so have we from our optimizing what is on our body for good reason-hair is protective, protecting the breast from toxins which are swept along and cleansed more easily with the underarm hair in tact doing what it does best, wick away toxins from the body.

You could consider it and become more comfortable with trimmed underarm hair instead of using yet more plastic shavers that go into the landfill and more aluminum based antiperspirant which is harmful to you. It causes your body to not perspire and detox under your arms and it also deposits white 'goo' under there are well. In my experience as a Massage Therapist it is just awful to reach under somebody's arm and get your fingers in that mess! You doing the detox in part or in whole you will notice that your body will not smell as much and you can more easily give up the more concealing armpit products that mask the smell under the arms, this will give your thyroid a break as well as your breast whether you are a male or a female.

## Body Washes

What about those body washes? Well, most of them sold in the stores are toxic and part of doing a detox to help yourself out and your thyroid gland is to become aware of what you are using and the ramifications of their continued use. Body washes are scented, most often unnaturally, you see, **fragrance oils and scents are far different from essential oil** based which is 'medicine.' Most commercial body wash and bubble bath has colorants, preservatives and shelf stabilizers. My personal preference is the

Nutribiotic Coconut Oil Soap in bulk in a bottle you can refill and add your own favorite essential oil to it. Locally, our small natural foods store sells it and you can bring in your own recycled bottle and buy as much as you like, use it plain, or, you can add some lavender to it to relax or peppermint essential oil which is invigorating, to help you to wakeup in the mornings!

Spacing out your showering to every other day, or every several days and sponge bathing becomes second nature once you try it, it just sounds odd at first. Same thing with underarms, I know from doing massage so many years that plenty of women forego shaving their legs in the winter and so we can adjust a bit in how we think and ease into making the changes you feel comfortable with that will benefit you and are more sustainable.

Just a note that If you live in the country or have well water, please, be sure to have your well water tested often, meaning at least every 2-3 years for arsenic, and other toxins in your water could adversely affect your health. I have had clients over the years who had problems with arsenic in their water. Any products that contain propyl gallate are to be avoided.

### Body Fragrance, Perfumes, Colognes and Body Sprays

Ever notice how when we spray a fragrance on the body we tend to aim right at the throat and near the thyroid gland? And, when we use fragrances, colognes, most perfumes, and body sprays they are loaded with toxic ingredients that can harm the thyroid gland, especially, if they are sprayed right onto it!

Instead, make your own healing mists and body sprays by getting some of your favorite essential oils, and this is for men as well as women and children! Use pure lavender essential oil, rosemary is a great tonic for our thyroid gland and mix the two in a spray bottle with water so that you are upgrading out of synthetic fragrance and into something beneficial for body, mind and spirit! You can make a body spray that is essential oil based with distilled water, a spray bottle and about 40 drops of just one single note oil like Lavender or mix a few like Lavender & Rosemary, or Vetiver and Sandalwood, Rose & Sage, or Ylang Ylang is another relaxing favorite. Upgrade from chemical products and help the body with essential oils like Rosemary that could also be brushed into the hair or a few drops on the skin brush in the morning to fresh up and help your thyroid gland with movement of the lymph fluids, moving congestion and rosemary for medicine.

You can have a lot of fun with essential oils and making healing misters and, even give them as gifts, they are sustainable and healthy for everyone! Rosemary essential oil is a great tonic for thyroid imbalances so be sure to pick up some and even put a few drops in your palm and lightly into your hair before you leave out the door for your day and it helps hair growth and keeps you balanced.

## Walking

Walking is one of my favorite things to do! Especially on a warm morning with birds singing, near a lake, creek or the ocean. To experience the morning dew on the greens and flowers, and see the bees, birds and their songs, and bird calls, the various animals.

When you walk you are stimulating the many reflex points that correlate with the organs of the body, the heart, lungs, pancreas, and all benefit from walking! You are stimulating these points and, at the same time, provided you have comfortable shoes with plenty of room for your entire foot that is not cramped up, and with a bendable footwear, you are stimulating your digestion so that you help move along material hanging out in your intestines. You help to clear your gallbladder, liver, and kidneys too! Remember, that your skin is one of your largest detoxification organs and you are helping your skin to breathe and detox as well just getting outside and moving your body and absorbing the fresh air, relaxing the mind out in Nature. Walking also helps to fire up your burners and get your temperature up a bit so if you are hypothyroid and cold all the time you will enjoy the warming sensation of a nice long walk. Please make sure to include this vital aspect in your plan to detox and heal your thyroid.

## Yoga

I don't know about you, but I do not always have time in the morning to do an hour of yoga on a yoga mat and then get the walk in with the dogs. I want to be able to make a juice, or a blended drink later after my brief yoga and walk. In the interest of time, I often combine my yoga with my morning walk. Meaning, that I bring a bag along and my yoga becomes bending and picking up trash on the walk along the river trail. In this way the dogs get out, I get sunshine on the body, fresh air, walking, and, yoga. The bending, reaching, and the way I use my body to get the trash I typically find at the Scanlon River Trails: vodka bottles, broken glass and cigarette butts left on the ground become my morning yoga many days! It's a Tri-Yoga experience: walking, cleaning and yoga! In an hour I am accomplishing getting the dogs out as well as contributing to the community, so, it works well for me! Where I usually go there is a deck overlooking the St. Louis River and I can utilize that sunny spot to do a few poses that I want to focus on, or a Sun Salutation and that works well too!

If you want another way to appreciate living somewhere that has the full expression of seasons, your winter mornings are ideal to get your mat out and use a DVD or some poses you feel good with, or stop at a class at the yoga studio or the local gym, or do some yoga with a friend.

In any event, I wanted to mention that it's not always formal yoga, but the breath, the **release of tension** to the muscles is very important. If we change how we express what we are aiming for from "stretching" to "releasing" tension, then our yoga need not be fancy to achieve what we are doing: breath, relaxation, oxygen to the blood, muscles and strengthening the bones are our goals! Yoga is about massaging your internal organs; even just seated floor poses like gentle spinal twists, plank pose, child's pose, mummy pose with a sandbag all facilitate better breathing, flexibility and strength.

### Sleep

This is a very important for healing your thyroid gland. You absolutely need to have a recharge time. Yet what is often left out today of our understanding of how to heal ourselves is when to get to sleep! People often relate with me that they just do better by staying up late and sleeping in later in the day. I have to disagree based upon what I learned from an Ayurveda Instructor, Cynthia Copple who taught a class about healing with Ayurveda and about our Ojas; our vital essence and how we deplete it by not sleeping with the Moon - ideally getting to sleep by 10pm and waking after 5 or 6 am to the Sun.

When it gets dark all animals know it is time to bed down and prepare to sleep and be quiet, except for humans. What distracts us most often aside from the many enticing screens, is that we often get a second wind, a burst of energy once we stay up past 10pm.

We will sleep much better if we avoid eating and most of our water and drinks within hours of planning to sleep. This way we are also not using energy to rejuvenate with the energy need to digest. Ever notice how the later you eat in the evening, and, before sleeping the hungrier you feel in the morning? I do! People stomach as "empty" and needing breakfast but with a little redirecting we can allay consuming calories a bit longer and have more energy and focus for the early part of our day. Taming the ways that we eat is beneficial for sleep.

So that you can ideally release melatonin and optimize your hormones we sleep in a dark room without light, nightlight, or a television-no blue screens of any kind, including laptops on the bed or screen light while you sleep. If you can, place them in another room or far away as possible when it's time to sleep. These are habits that confuse the brain that is geared to sleep in a dark space. It is best to remove televisions from any bedroom that you or your children sleep in as they emit radiation and listening to news and then going to sleep will produce a less rested sleep if the mind is preoccupied with negativity. You can trim some of the news watching in the same way we ask young people to reduce some of the social media for their own persona wellness.

I have often related about the off gassing factors to consider when sleeping on many of our beds including tempur-pedic and memory foam types beds being some of the worst, and also carpeting, couches, chairs, linoleum and more. Probably your best choice is an organic cotton futon, or, sleeping on the floor, of the Earth and even camping in a tent for some people.

## Congestive Sleep Apnea

People who have **congestive sleep apnea** can easily use this book to clear congestion and release the need for a machine to sleep at night, it may take a little bit of time but it will happen most of the time once you remove the congestion and build upon the lifestyle habits. A part of congestive issues that cause sleep apnea are the inflammation that cause restriction and problems breathing. Many people reduce or eliminate snoring, sleep apnea, and other sleep problems by detoxification and healing as outlined for their thyroid in this book.

## Cleaners

Household cleaners and commercial cleaners need to be rethought and upgraded as part of your detox and heal plan. Many people just buy the same thing and feel like cleaning is not really clean if they do not smell that pine or other scent that they have become used to. Did you know you can make your own cleaner with a spray bottle and essential oils, or vinegar and there are many ways to make non-toxic cleaners that you can add pine or lemon essential oils that will not be toxic.

At the gym I formerly belonged to they sprayed cleaner on other machines while we worked out that was completely toxic. When I mentioned to them that I would rather have an occasional bacteria as opposed to harmful toxins used in high strength cleaners that I would never use in my own home, they looked dumbfounded? I don't get it?

If you are still using a cleaner that is pink, orange or something like Pine Sol, please, take a moment and realize that this is not the end all of cleaners, this stuff is toxic.

## Animals

Many of us live with companion or service animals and we love them! They are part of our family and again, as part of your detox and heal plan, you need to take a look at what is being used on your companions on many levels. Often times Veterinarians recommend products I would absolutely never use. People want to be good citizens and follow the rules and do right by their dogs, cats, and other animals they live with and take good care of them, but, many of the items that most people get are causing both you and the animal to be exposed to some serious chemicals.

Many of the flea, tick, worming and other products many people use for help with pests and their companions are also very toxic to your thyroid gland as well as to the being you share space with. Please consider investigating other options that are non-toxic and saving yourself the exposure as well.

I often guide people into using the same DE and clays for their animal companions which if given regularly to a healthy animal who does not live on kibble (dry food) exclusively will work just fine.

## Air Fresheners

Many people use Glade and other super toxic air "fresheners" which really means toxic products that change the smell of the air transforming it with chemicals that are harmful to your lungs, throat and your thyroid gland.

Essential oils made into a healing mister work very well as well as on cotton balls and placed around the home or diffused into the air.

Look at your candles as well as many are very toxic to breathe in on a regular basis with colorants, chemicals and artificial fragrances.

## Detox & Pain

Did you know that we have alternatives to using many of our commercial pain relievers for headaches, joint pain, and general aches and pain.

In the same way that people think nothing of using a Spray and Wash bottle to spray stains and then throw their laundry into the washing machine, when a brush and a bit of soap will do we can often detoxify and prevent most of the perceived need for NSAID use.

Becoming more hydrated, walking, getting to sleep earlier, reducing our calories, eating more healthfully and doing many of the detoxification steps listed in this book will reduce the need for over the counter pain medications. Reduce inflammation and joint swelling and for sure, headaches and migraines. We are reducing the toxic load of our cells. This liberates us financially from buying more of these, saves our liver and kidneys and makes us more productive people often in a better mood.

People use other remedies for the occasional pain management, which occurs with less frequency when you upgrade yourself after a detox. White willow bark which can be ingested as herbal capsules, or, smoked works pretty well and was the original aspirin. We have herbs that when used as tea on a regular basis like nettle leaf tea, that help the body to remineralize.

We have the ability to truly look at our lives from the perspective of how can we make things more simple, less toxic, and less inflammation and pain by procuring good daily habits. It takes 5-10 minutes to make a blend-ed cantaloupe drink and out the door you go with a great tasting drink that gets your through the morning and serves up nutrients, a serving of fruit, or two, if you include what I do on occasion and blend in a frozen organic banana or two. Strawberries, and banana, or acai berry and banana, helps you to begin to replace yogurts made from dairy products that is often added and replace it with coconut kefir or almond yogurt, coconut water or milk and you have a great blended smoothie, or acai bowl that you can make and take out the door with you if you are heading to work or school.

With detoxification, if you have consumed the Standard American Diet ("SAD"), most of your life it will take a bit of time for your body to release the excess weight, inflammation; it leaves via your bowel movements, urine and sweat. For stomach upsets which can happen, I highly recommend L Glutamine, which can be opened as a capsule and emptied on the tongue or sublingual as well as swallowed. L Glutamine is a non essential amino acid that aids in recovery of your immune system so instead of using over-the-counter products for stomach distress, loose bowels, and tanked immune function, turn to L Glutamine which also helps your glutathione levels as well!

You will know when you get closer to health as you no longer have a plugged nose, sneezing every morning when you reduce the sugar intake and the crusty eyes, the mucous draining from your nose in the shower or sauna. You will no longer sit in the bathroom for 5-30 minutes and destroy your toilet as well as go through scads of toilet paper! And, the bathroom will not smell like a crusty colon.

Given the amount of sales of "Poop Spray" that is something used for our restrooms because people leave behind an awful smell is proclamation that we stink! Thousands of spray bottles of poop spray are sold through Groupon and other sales sites online, websites and all over! What you place in your mouth and through lifestyle products affects your smell, under your arms, your yoni, your anus, bowel movements, and your perspiration will either smell like herbs, flowers, and fruits, vegetables, or, it will smell like rotting and mucous which does not smell very good. In fact, most people do not realize that when they leave the restroom it smells horrible, just their urine alone!

When you are detoxed, you will understand and living amongst people who never detoxify or need longer time to detoxify and then they keep dip-ping into the sugar and processed foods, will sneeze in the morning and blame it on "allergies."

Once your body is cleaned out, the organs functioning and your glands, especially your thyroid gland, you will no longer smell awful and there will be no need to cover anything up except for the occasional choice you make and you will immediately sense and smell what you consumed whether a coffee drink, alcohol, nitrates, dairy, or wheat, you will sense immediately or by the next morning, the crust in the corners of your eyes, your urine and bowel movements will smell and your underarms will wreak! This is probably why it became so fashionable to shave the underarms in the first place is because that horrid smell lingers onto the hairs that are there to cleanse your lymph nodes under your arms.

You see, over the years, people ask me to target healing their liver, or their cancer in a certain area, or their thyroid gland. We cannot just focus on entirely your thyroid gland. We cannot remove it and repair it. We can cause your body to heal from the inside the way it does naturally, which is allow it to downsize the load of weight, mucous, congestion, stagnation, and then feed it nutrients, vitamins, enzymes, minerals, give it sleep, respite from the sea of signals all around us amping up our nervous system, heart and brain.

We have choices, we can remove ourselves if we are in toxic and stressful relationships, jobs, businesses, if we spend time around toxic people who refuse to change, they are sullen, upset, negative, just exit, it is our own choice. Even if it takes you some time, make a plan so that you can remove yourself from any of those scenarios. It could be where you live and that you just are not happy or at peace with yourself, so be honest. Do you go to functions even though you do not want to? Begin to detox and through this process, begin to become more of a direct communicator. What is direct? It is not blunt, it is not judgmental, or rude, it means you can be kind and at the same time you can make your requests known, or, you can keep them to yourself and have a plan to transition yourself from the person who is so low vibration and toxic over a period of time with resources you plan to gather. Find a new church, friends, partner, job, whatever it is, do not let it cause you to compromise your quality of life.

**One thorn of experience is worth a whole wilderness of warning - James Russell Lowell**

# CHAPTER TEN - DETOX & MIND BODY MEDICINE

Mind Body Medicine also known as 'Psychosomatics,' is rarely understood as fully as it could be applied today. Reason being is that people wanted to be absolved of their own personal responsibility for their state of health. Mind Body medicine looks at the symbolic ways our body evidences what is happening in our mind; your unconscious mind stores many memories that often reproduce like a ripple from experiences you once had or you expect to have in the future. What Mind Body can show us is the symbolic roadmap based upon our experiences, diseases, accidents and more. It is an important tool in terms of wellness and understanding what our mind creates. It is also a great tool for releasing programs in the mind.

Thyroid imbalances are often associated with humiliation and there is no shortage of this feeling today, just look at stressors that affect people today, including the cost of life and other stressors we deal with today. People feel stressed hearing about the government, the world leaders, their jobs, businesses, and the state of the Earth and the environment.

You will begin to notice that large segments of people in the world end up experiencing the same disease, conditions or syndromes. As I shared earlier thyroid has a component of feeling choked or humiliated. People talk about throat chakra energy and how this relates with your neck and thyroid with feeing heard, or having a voice in life.

Mind Body Medicine is my number one tool I use to find the origin of lack of ease somebody is carrying within them-within the mind and now, manifesting in the body, mentally, emotionally or spiritually. What I find is quite surprising and I do not need to assume the role of the psychologist or analyst to consult with anyone about what is coming up in their lives.

I listen to their story; I note key words, where and when, how and hear the story but I also keenly observe the body language, the face, lips, eyes, skin, if possible, their walk and when I take people out to Nature to "pack up," I am very aware of their footing, how they are balanced as well as their speech, is it rapid, staggered, staccato, rigid, stoic, you can deeply listen to the inflection of the tone, the throat clearing, as well as watch where the arms will guard key parts of the body. If you know a bit about basic reading of body language that is a part of it. I have adapted to the use of Mind Body medicine to use it over the course of helping someone much like coaches do in my consulting where I can guide their language, breathing, and give them specific ideas about releasing long held pain. *Each person has aspects of Mind that are producing internal dialogue and thoughts if we do not tend to them, our garden becomes unhealthy.*

And, I believe that if we had people trained with these ways that I work with people we would have dramatically lower "Health Care Costs" and fewer people on machines, in hospital beds, drugged and cut open. People helping others in the way of Original Medicine would guide people with the many ways I am sharing with you in this book and there are more.

Mind Body Medicine could be better understood today. Mention Mind Body Medicine to most people and likely they will expect some form of relaxation: taking a retreat with a yoga mat and perhaps a guided meditation. Certainly this is a small part of Mind Body Medicine also known as Psychosomatics but there is much more to this that was removed from our current forms of medicine today.

Without the use of Original Medicine, and, detoxification as a primary means of restoring homeostasis, we often omit the obvious remedies. Take for example the use the word "disorder," which presents and feels like a broken machine. Many a Disorder contains symptoms that are very much aligned with Dr. Sarno's remarkable tension-myositis-syndrome. Dr. Sarno, MD, speaks to these common experiences of pain that people experience and how they are produced by the mind-symptoms disappear when the mind is released. How do we get the mind released, especially if we have tension responses to long held memories even from childhood? Walking, and yoga, which release tension from the mind.

Our current medical industry has a very codified and unified system. Many people will quickly correct you in a very legalistic way if you take healing into your own head, heart and hands and restore your homeostasis. While many people are eager to heal themselves, others are far removed from trusting their self and they do not know where to begin. The paradigm is heavily enforced with historical movements and memories where people were punished for failure to obey and conform; people want to be good.

There is a Mind Body component for each and every problem that arises, every symptom. In the 1800s many psychologists were studying psychosomatics which is the original name for Mind Body Medicine meaning that the mind, and more specifically, our thoughts, influence what happens with our 'soma' our body. Mind Body Medicine is very easy to understand once you really understand how our unconscious and subconscious mind hold on to memories at a young age when we did not have the ability to filter out our experiences and how we are experiencing the world today, day by day reacting to what we experience. As Dr. John Sarno, MD writes in his book The Divided Mind, we end up with tension syndromes he calls "TMS" that are produced as the mind is tense and the body has **diminished blood and oxygen flow to key areas of the body**. I have a couple of courses on Mind Body Medicine in general and one specifically geared to Thyroid issues. I began an interest in 1984 in Mind Body and at first, I'll be candid, I felt it was pretty 'airy' however, as I came to use it more and more and gain a proficient understanding as well as explored what some of our many respected psychoanalysts like Alfred Adler, Carl Jung, Sigmund Freud and others had to say, as well as found the way it worked for myself and then for clients, over 30 years later now I find it my number one go to. Mind Body is how I 'map' what is happening with a client because if we merely 'treat' people with drugs, surgeries, and radiation, or chemotherapy, while they are warranted in trauma and relatively few comparative situations to how we use them today, as I see it we have a bit of a dependency on being "treated," we can get to the actual root and our pain and syndromes and symptoms becomes a way to balance. I use Mind Body Medicine, Nutrition, Herbs, Massage, releasing tension from the body with walking and yoga, sleep, restoring our connection with Nature by encouraging diurnal balance.

### Cysts, Nodules & Tumors

Years ago my eyes were opened wide when I read Dr. Brownstein's works and he stated about cysts, nodules and tumors. It really clicked for me after over a decade of giving massage and wellness work in Minnesota— **most of my clients had so many cysts that I could easily palpate during a massage treatment.** I related this with clients many times each week about the cysts under their arms, armpit area, along their clavicle, around their neck and in many places, but the largest proportion of cysts was on the breast near the areola: the nipple. As a therapist, we are not massaging the breast, but when clients had extensive cysts, I would ask them to place their fingers across their clavicle and then on the very sides of their breast using the sheet on top and showing them how to feel for the lumps, bumps and small round cysts that had collected there and why detoxification: diet, walking and more would greatly prevent the certain issues that would come from the cysts collecting in the body.

Cysts form in many places in the body. At one time, we formerly had from fresh spring water, and a clean high mineral food source from the Earth. Cysts form in predictable areas of the body as well that are lacking in iodine. They show up as cysts on the follicles of the ovaries, in the uterus as fibroids, and, in the breasts as Fibro-Cystic Breast Disease, as Breast Cancer, as Uterine Cancer, as Ovarian Cancer and, often Fibromyalgia is discussed as having "trigger points" points of pain which is also a byproduct of fibrin which is produced in more abundance due to our diet, our lack of movement, our stress, and our lack of sufficient Iodine. **Massage Therapy is an excellent medicine** to use for helping you to detox as well as help facilitate lymphatic and blood flow, increase oxygen to your cells, and particularly if you are unable to exercise as much as the therapist is manually moving your fluids for you similar to you getting out and exercising although not entirely the same.

**Sauna is also a great way to help your detoxing from the cysts,** nodules and some tumors. As we discussed about wheat, and it's congesting properties, and dairy it's congealing effects and depositing excess calcium which offsets your minerals as discussed by Dr. Thompson in his book The Calcium Lie 2, this sort of calcium and too much of it offsets your magnesium and other minerals. Many people like my paternal grandmother having absorbed the marketing of our needing calcium and protein faithfully got lots of calcium and women for many generations faithfully as well took calcium supplements despite the body showing signs that this was harming them with their fingernails and skin.

A cyst which continues to accumulate congesting and congealing, and a person who is now moody and does not apply daily habits of love and success and get out and walk in Nature, get to the gym, do some yoga, release tension will begin to cause more problems, perhaps forming into a **nodules** as it would upon your thyroid gland on the follicles just as PCOS does on the follicles on your ovaries. What is you knew that detoxification the ways that I show you in this book truly work to reduce these cysts, eliminate them and then the use of the minerals will keep you as well as removing the foods we discuss in this book will have you feeling much better and preventing instead of having the cysts 'medicated,' or cut out with surgery, or the use of ablations. Doctors know that many people will not change and so they are rather forced to have procedures for people so that they do the work for them. Please do not interpret me as saying that everyone is just taking this route, I surely am not saying this, I am saying that I have worked on people and with them for shoulder impingements that could have been worked out with time and changing daily habits and I related this with scores of clients who simply declined and went the route of shoulder surgeries, rotator cuff surgeries and continued to eat wheat, dairy, factory farmed meat, nitrate lunch meats, high sugars, and not exercise and so the way of the healthcare industry today is to remove the fault of the patient and place the burden upon the Doctor to fix us and that too, is in defense of our precious Doctors clearly unfair.

Why not find a solution and not just a bandaid? Instead of just drugging, cutting and killing, battling it out of people, fighting it, **why not educate and put the money that we spend drugging people into zombies, into education and food forests?** Just the money we spent on one political election is enough to feed the entire United States by distributing heirloom seeds, cleaning up our water together and getting our cells back in balance.

Our body must be cared for, or, **in defense it forms cysts**, and if the warnings are not heeded nodules that are hardened, and then, tumors. If you do not feed your cells and provide ample minerals: magnesium, iodine, selenium, copper, chromium and more, you will lose bone, muscle, connective tissue, myelin, and your cell membrane will not conduct electricity as well; your plasma will not be as healthy as the vital conductor of electricity for you and you will get that check engine light of anxiety, disturbed moods, lack of energy and cysts.

The first part of the detox in preparing with probiotic, clay or DE, skin brushing is extremely beneficial for helping you to reduce and eliminate your cysts, nodules and tumors. You have likely heard of many people learning that they have benign tumors in their head and this like **breast cancer has shown great response with high doses of iodine.**(Supervised only)

Massage Therapy treatments, sauna, walking, using the first part of detox will help you to reduce and eliminate cysts and nodules so that your body can restore homeostatic balance. You, know what you need to do to rebalance yourself, you just needed the reminder-the guidance.

When you detox and heal you will begin shedding pounds of pain, mucous, congestion, mucous in the head, parasites, candida, and you will heal in profound ways.

Iodine detoxifies your organs and, it shrinks the masses!

You can talk about how dangerous iodine is all day and I will still say that whether somebody is hyperthyroid or hypothyroid once they detox a bit, get walking and make some changes they can tolerate it just fine especially in smaller doses. Thyroid hormones are in large part made from it. This is just common sense, and with big thanks to Dr. Brownstein, MD.

### Radiation

Some radiation is harmful and can even be the cause of thyroid cancer. Such is the case for people who were exposed to nuclear experiments throughout time in Nevada and elsewhere.

**Wikipedia** states this about ionizing radiation:

"...thyroid cancer, often occurs when nuclear weapons and reactors are the radiation source because of the biological proclivities of the radioactive iodine fission product, iodine-131.[3] However, calculating the exact risk and chance of cancer forming in cells caused by ionizing radiation is still not well understood..."

The developing baby in utero was the most affected by exposures to I 131 radiation. I have to wonder why we allowed these experiments to be conducted for so many years in Nevada, as well as Marshall Islands. We also have Fukushima and Chernobyl to think about with regard to radiation and our health.

Thyroid issues show up in many ways, some websites state at least 300 symptoms that are common to thyroid imbalance, like **Hypothyroid Mom**. I know from much experience that far too many young people are not able to deal with the anxiety they suffer from, which seemed odd to me at first, but I studied it and I see why.

First, the wheat situation; the factory farmed animals and their anxiety, all the sugar we consume, and the helpless way we feel when we are over-whelmed with the world-as if we are grasped by the throat. **Generalized Anxiety Disorder**, "GAD," could be helped by healing the whole person, and not seeing it as a separate and distinct syndrome from the body giving us a red flag that something is not right. Anxiety is creating the future recluse of tomorrow at a far younger age than ever before known. GAD is completely reversible.

Our young people will continue to suffer with anxiety and depression, as well as sleeping issues without the proper help; and that help is not a drug, perhaps temporarily as a stop gap, but not in the long run-it's detoxification. People are often magnesium deficient, and, they have gut issues from a life-time of eating grains, including wheat, cheese, meats, nitrates, soft drinks, and energy drinks, they have **gut rot** and often other gut issues that must be repaired which I believe holds a brighter promise to heal and rejuvenate a person than to medicate for the remainder of their life. Healing the gut, adding magnesium and then checking on the thyroid with a simply ultra-sound as well as HTMA (hair tissue mineral analysis), and BBTs (basal body temperatures). First, heal the gut including using probiotics and clarify the diet, add in the magnesium and then begin to do the work if necessary on balancing the thyroid gland.

**Can you detoxify your body from radiation?** Yes, you can, most often using Earth! You can also use the **chlorophyll** of green leafy plants and **chlorella and spirulina** in tablets or powder in smoothies. Chlorella is a powerful detoxifier and noted as the claw action detoxifier for the body, grabbing toxins to help pull them from the body. I have often bought spir-ulina, and chlorella at ultimate superfoods through their online store.

To use **Earth**: You would use clay, like Bentonite, Redmond, and other clays, and Earth & Water like Diatomaceous Earth "DE" and you use it daily to pull the toxins and radiation from the body and eliminate it through the bowel and the sweat. You can decide which one you use or try one of each and begin by adding a teaspoon to your water in the morning a half hour before your probiotic, or an hour after so it does not grab and use up your probiotic and you could also use it at other times during the day.

We do not even think about radiation, yet, it's all around us, everywhere! Cell phones, electrical magnetic fields, "EMFs," our refrigerators, tv, appliances, laptops, modems, and more. The less exposure the better, thus we want to keep exposure to a minimum; not carry our phones on our body, clipped to our hip and with bluetooth appliances on and near our heads. I have often observed women placing their cell phones into their bra or in their head wrap with the cell phone inside positioned against their ear holding a conversation. These devices are seeking a signal to operate and they produce heat that can permeate our skull, our breast, and affect our glands, including our thyroid gland. These cell phones that nearly all of us have in our hands are capable of reducing your TSH - thyroid stimulating hormone levels. Radiation is essentially *cooking* the cysts, nodules and tumors in your body, and in your brain.

What is gene mutation and how does a gene become mutated? Ionizing radiation can mutate genes and so does exposure to many drugs, chemical agents, DDT, and halides like chlorine, fluoride, and bromine.

# CHAPTER ELEVEN - IODINE & SUPPLEMENTS

You need **iodine** to make up a few of your thyroid hormones and most people are deficient in iodine. T3 is three parts iodine and T4 is four parts iodine. For some reason, iodine was removed from many of our foods where it was used as a preservative. Toxic halides were added like bromine as a dough conditioner. Halides compete for space on your thyroid where iodine would be in the follicles and they can weaken your thyroid in instances like with fluoride which was used for this purpose-to slow the thyroid in years past.

**Most people do well with 12.5 mg of iodine to start**. I began on a small transdermal dose, then increased to 12.5 mg, and I now take 50mg per day for several weeks and then I take about a week break on supplements. I also consume molecular iodine in the form of kelp, Nori, and other seaweeds.

Iodine is a major detoxifier and it is needed by every cell in your body. Your thyroid gland needs iodine to function. If you have more of an interest, please read Dr. Brownstein's book on Iodine.

## Magnesium

Magnesium Glycinate releasing tension, relaxes, making protein, bone, muscle, blood pressure, blood sugar, and your DNA. Early signs of magnesium deficiency include loss of appetite, nausea, vomiting, fatigue, and weakness. As magnesium deficiency worsens, numbness, tingling, muscle contractions and cramps, seizures, personality changes, abnormal heart rhythms, and coronary spasms can occur. Just about everyone today needs to supplement with magnesium.

**Selenium** is a mineral that assists with thyroid with iodine, and also detoxification of mercury, it helps to detoxify the brain. Most people recommend 200 mcg. It is important to supplement with selenium especially if you are taking iodine.

### Tyrosine (L Tyrosine)

Tyrosine is very important for thyroid health and helps to facilitate iodine, however, I recommend that you check with somebody you are working with or your doctor to make sure this would work well for you.

### Iodine

So many people, including doctors are unsure and afraid of iodine. We have to have iodine and I can share with you that I have greatly benefited from it, I am glad I chose to use it. Some people have some brief and mild detox experiences from iodine like skin rashes or some stomach upset, but, I have to say that these are more common with people who did not detox first. Please, detox first!

### Detox first!

Ok, so there are many products online you can choose from, many are too low in iodine to do any real major healing and at first most people will be afraid of iodine so research it for yourself so you feel more comfortable. Don't just listen to anybody, look it up, and be sure.

There are nascent types at Global Healing online that I have tried and liked very much and as of now, I use Iodoral and I take the 50 mg supplement daily, and, I take Tyrosine 500 mg and I also take selenium 200-400 micrograms.

For many years I sold a Lugol's solution transdermal that you apply to the skin with a dropper and I showed clients how to use it on their forearms or wherever they wish to apply it, but that is a low dose compared to a therapeutic dose like I am taking now, just know that there are many options, I started out slow and you might want to also to be sure you feel comfortable and safe.

I have read in some of the books I read that some doctors take 75 mg every day because it is a protective element and thyroid imbalances are associated with a great many health problems. Iodine needed by the body and there is a lot written that you can read about how without it, many people have been born mentally retarded, and our body cannot function properly without this element particularly because of the amount of bromide we are exposed to today that our body needs to detoxify from in the drinks as BVO and in brominated flour that makes up most of our breads and other wheat items sold as food, in body products and lots more!

I have read several books on iodine and, I highly recommend Dr. Brownstein's book on Iodine if you are seeking more information.

## Vitamin C

One of the fastest ways to plump up the cells of the body and heal quickly, as well as help to heal your thyroid is to have vitamin C every day. I like the food based product known as Pure Radiance by Synergy Company which has a variety of berries and acerola cherry powder.

You can get powder or capsules and I prefer the powder so that I can easily mix it with water or in a cold blended drink and often it is recommended to use 3 grams per day in 3-1 gram doses. The thing about Vitamin C is that if you do too much for you the only problem is that your stools will become lose and you can back off a bit.

## Zinc

Zinc helps your immune system and your hormone production. It is an anti inflammatory, helps with hair loss, Chronic Fatigue Syndrome, and nerve dysfunction as well as your gut. People usually suck on zinc lozenges when they first feel a cold coming on and zinc is very helpful. I like the liquid zinc that you can add to your water along with vitamin C powder by Synergy as they go well together and there is very little taste to this liquid zinc. Eidon Minerals make a liquid zinc but there are other brands and other ways to take zinc as well.

For people who are high copper zinc is absolutely critical and it will bring down the mania of fast talking, super busy mind that a high copper personality can manifest, including their intensity and feeling easily distracted. Can you imagine now, how many problems could be solved by identifying mineral deficiencies and excesses, restoring balance to mineral depletion and lack and correcting mineral and heavy metal excesses in the body? We can do great things! And, minerals are replenishing where medications often have side effects we wish to avoid.

Once you have your hair tissue mineral analysis you can review what minerals and metals, foods and know your metabolic type so that you can more accurately hone in on repairing your thyroid and get the right mix of supplements. After you detox and review your report you can get to healing your thyroid most often, quite easily.

**ZINC RICH PUMPKIN SEED MILK:** One of my favorite ways to get more zinc in my diet is to make fresh raw pumpkin seed milk. I take 1/4

- 1/2 cup of raw green pumpkin seeds and blend in my Blendtec blender with a blender 2/3 full of filtered water and a small pinch of iodized sea salt and sometimes I add a capful of pure organic vanilla, it is delicious! And, has lots of zinc!

# CHAPTER TWELVE - HEALING YOUR THYROID

Healing your thyroid will involve keeping your daily plan and your food diary, and I have an example of what that may look like, down below. You will need to focus an effort on reducing and eliminating carrying a burden with cysts, shrink any nodules and resolve tumors through detoxification.

Because of these multigenerational thyroid issues, not only am I seeing younger people that are loaded with cysts, under their arms, around the breast, but also with lipoma or Buffalo Hump as well. Sadly, many people are unable to focus enough to read a book, and retain what they have read nor sustain focus to finish an entire book due to impulsivity due to the exposure to chemicals, from many of their habits like cigarette smoking, constant use of cannabis, lack of walking outdoors, and food chemicals.

When people are carrying a lot of mucous and waste they also have a very strained lymphatic system. Regenerating health is developing habits to stay well like walking, drinking filtered water, and, eating fresh real food.

Cannabis is a wonderful medicine it truly is, however, I see people smoking every single day and often throughout the day vaping, dabbing, and using this as a coping mechanism. We have other options like amino acids and remineralization of the body which will help to calm so that you are not vaping and smoking all day long. I really appreciate cannabis as a medicine but, I also want to be able to see people enjoying their lives separate from using constantly. **People are eating far too much and too often, the toilet, nor their eyes do not lie.**

We spend too much time sitting and watching screens and as a result our skin just has no vibrance or shine to it. Our schools are not teaching people how to take care of your own body and to heal they are reinforcing the dominant programs by requiring vaccines and physical exams because that is what most people know.

I have seen many high school students and young adults in consultation and speaking with them at my home when my son lived with me, that were under 25 and I have serious concerns because of their levels of anxiety, sexual fetish, and hormonal problems. While they have money to get their nails and hair done, or order expensive brands like True Religion, they do not have common sense about how to thrive and stay healthy. It is my belief that all of the ADHD, ODD and learning disabilities are preventable and that we can reverse most of the ADHD and ODD and greatly help the learning disabled. But we have to start!

If we remain linear, resistant and rigid which is what happens on a starch stiff diet, one that is too high in chemicals and requires detoxification as we will do in this book to cause our own thyroid gland to reboot, we need change: real change! Your diet has everything to do with your mental flexibility, your speed of thought and your ability to think outside the box. If you are swollen in the face, body, legs, and you have not found how to detox, please, do this and do yourself a favor you will be thankful you did. Many of the predicable ways we think of aging are just not true-you do not have to go down a predictable path. Upgrade yourself and live long so you can enjoy your retirement.

### Thyroid & Sexual Issues

Glandular problems including thyroid and adrenal can produce some odd behaviors emotionally, mentally and sexually. Thyroid problems can vacillate between slow and fast or hypo and hyper depending on the status of your thyroid and how exhausted your adrenal glands become. I have had years to figure out a plan or set of ways I can respond for a client when they or, somebody else calls for them asking for a consult to help to calm down their thyroid. We first seek to calm and then to restore. To restore, we need to do follow up consults with some hand holding through a detox so that instead of finding the medication to be on forever and burying the problems they begin to remove the symptoms and reverse the problem from the root.

I will share that Amino acids work really well for temporary use and, they are brain food. Next, minerals that bring calm to the central nervous system heart and brain, and as soon as possible, I want to start reducing those cysts. **It is my opinion that people also have these cysts in the brain** and in many places. That they are almost 'baked' by way of the EMF and radiation exposures and that we further congest and congeal them by continuing our poor habits that nearly all of us were programmed with: dairy and wheat. **Many of our behaviors are closeted until enough people become comfortable with them.** Important to note is that with all the cysts and lumps, bumps, cysts and nodules, tumors in the body and brain they can and do interfere with the brain and they can be part of why we see some abnormal behaviors, sexually and otherwise. We also see flat affect and sullen, toxic moods, low energy, low vibrance and a paste like look in many young adults. I have done my best to "sneak" in the chlorophyll which is different from taking a pill or supplement that is chlorophyll it is not the same as plants which received sunlight energy.

I have personal knowledge through being a local healer in a small city that **many young people have extreme and odd sexual fetishes and behaviors and, that hyperthyroid produces a very strong hyper sexuality with risky behaviors.** They are risky because they can also potentially injure an unsuspecting partner which was the case for one of my clients whose husband was venturing out to meet up and have unprotected sex without any protection nor information exchanged.

In addition to meeting with 12-16 year olds with their parents or grandparent and hearing directly from them that they look in the mirror in the morning and wonder if they should kill themselves to also hearing from others that they masturbate and need sex several times per day. Do you see what we are doing to ourselves? And, to our children?

I do. I live this and I see this every day. Not only do I live it and see it, massage it and offer consultations, I study, read, gather, get out in nature and ask, "what can I do?" Having been a therapeutic foster parent for nearly 10 years I also saw odd behaviors but now with my experience level with the amount of success I have seen with myself and hundreds of people I have helped I realize there is something we can do about it, and drugging as maybe a very temporary stop gap but it is not our solution long term. We need to make changes. Large residential treatment centers need to change their diet plans and how they dispense medications, I have experience with this working with these agencies like Northwoods Children's Homes in Duluth, MN.

I also have experience being adrenal depleted and exhausted and thyroid imbalanced and I know what can happen for parents when next thing you know you look like a drug addict and you are screaming, ranting and raging. I brought myself back from this because I love my son and myself and I cared to do it naturally without medication. I also upgraded my brain from where I was and detoxed myself from all those heavy metal mercury amalgams and learned to balance my copper imbalance issues which produce moods as well. I know for sure I can help just about anybody reverse ADHD and ODD if given the time, meaning more than one session, it is a journey and we find the right combination of healing the mind and the diet so the person can regenerate their health. Truth be told most people today have some level of autism on the spectrum due to our way of life. Imagine if you felt good all the time? Flexible, could easily bend and touch your toes. Your toes, legs did not creak and crack and you were clear of thought and bright as the day? Would that be worth it to detox and heal? You will have to want this! Because you can read the book all you want but you have to do it and, it is not hard!

When your brain and hormones are not working well, like many people all over the world today, exposed to heavy metals, toxins and your body is toxic from halides and food chemicals, **you can expect very toxic behaviors: this, is what I am seeing and it is very disturbing.** I have parents of teens and young adults come talk with me about everything from wondering if their teen or young adult child is spiritually possessed to wondering what on earth to do when they have sent them to a local mental health hospital several times and it is not doing a thing for them.

Healing, means that people who are suffering, often our young people and have these thoughts of suicide and emotional, mental and sexual behaviors get some relief! We cannot just turn them all into zombies with drugs through the pharmacy or on the streets? And, when they mature enough and are fortunate enough to get off these drugs they have a heck of a mess to clean up from being out of their mind.

First calming the thyroid because it has been struggling for so long and then, we must begin to fuel the body with minerals and iodine, after we calmed them down. The doctors are still prescribing Ambien and they are also prescribing Klonopin for some of my client's children. When we are no longer here for our children they will be left with the repercussions of using these drugs long term and habituated into finding a drug to take away their pain. Most won't even entertain the idea of detoxification because mineral depletion turns them into very left brain dominant analytical and strictly practical types and they won't entertain anything that is not a linear solution very often.

I have experienced a great deal of young adults using drugs as a way to cope with the incessant pressures with anxiety and depression. One of the things I see with also doing the massage therapy for nearly 15 years were young people in their early 20s that do not eat vegetables, they do not exercise, they do a lot of drugs and they have some really odd habits, a combination of compulsive, sexual and habitual that many families are dealing with the best they can. Some of the wealthy put their young adult in their own home and others have just adapted the best that they can given the stress. I have at least 25 clients whose children had heroin problems and I relate that this particular drug creates a hero within "heroin." Sadly, these youth have been placed in front of the TV, bussed off the school early and most of them that I speak with had mothers who either took a medication from the doctor to dry up their milk and did not breastfeed as there was more toxic information about not breastfeeding, or not ruining their breasts so that their husbands would not be turned off? I don't know but I have heard it enough to feel pretty sad about it.

For several decades now we have witnessed hormonal changes that have happened to us as a result of eating factory farmed animals pumped with these chemicals, hormones and antibiotics that changed us and now, we have a lot of confusion. A lot of sexual, psychological and unfortunately, people that are very damaged; people that have been lost now to the onslaught of chemicals and hormones. I have had a lot of visits to the hospital for clients and their family and friends' family only to be shocked and dismayed at the involuntary intubating, drugging and mechanical way our precious people and elders are treated.

If I did not feel so absolutely sure that this, what is in this book, would be part of what would help us to make such a huge turn around, I would not have taken my time to write this book, nor would I have written it this way. I realize most people just want to get it over with and fix their thyroid gland and move on, but real healing doesn't work that way. We find ourselves right here, now which means I cannot walk my dogs where I usually go due to mercury and dioxin contamination in our rivers and there are laws mandating certain behaviors that I personally do not subscribe to, but they are invented each day as a "response," to the insanity, we need to deal with the root cause and our thyroid is an invitation to do so.

People were and still are damaged by radiation, by chemicals, by mineral deficient soils that grow our foods. They are full of waste that they need to detox out of their body to reinstate their glands so that they function again. Bromide which is a halogen is a large contributor to the sluggish thyroid and taking the place of where iodine would go in the thyroid gland. Bromide is in everything! The drinks I spoke of earlier, as BVO, and bromide is in lotions, body products, and the largest chunk of it has been in our wheat items like breads, muffins, and so in addition to the wheat itself you have the brominated flour which is done as a dough conditioner to expedite the process. Never before in history have we brushed our teeth with fluoride, rinsed our mouth with chlorine and fluoride, showered in it, ate fake foods, wheat and brominated flours, had drinks that were brominated, artificially colored and in aluminum cans and we are prescribed way more medications which have numerous and untold side effects particularly in combinations never before explored.

**When another person uses this book to detoxify and makes the conscious choice to eat and live clean allowing their body to be slim and healthy and functioning well, they are another model worthy of imitation and eventually we reach critical mass;** at the start we influence a great deal from grocery stores, to collective community gardens, to changing school food programs.

Please, get your composition books at the dollar store, label one of them your daily plan and the other your food diary. Get your probiotic, skin brush, clay and DE, and any supplements noted in your plan. Decide if you will order a general cleanse to get your elimination channels cleaned out a bit and order that or find it at your local natural foods store.

Now, you're ready to note in your plan on the first page, your first day: Just write in Day One and write down:

**Day One *Example* in Your Composition Book**

Wake up and Give Thanks!
Take my probiotic and drink some filtered water
Do some light skin brushing and, find a good place in my room or bathroom so I always see it!

Make a juice or blended drink, add in vitamin C powder and liquid zinc
Take a 5HTP if you have a lot of anxiety
Eat fresh fruit

Order my Supplements and/or cleanse package
Make sure I have filtered water
Have dark leafy greens (chlorophyll is highly healing and detoxing) as a part of your meal, in a salad, or blended in a green smoothie

Order an HTMA to start and get clear on my heavy metal exposure, minerals, nutritional profile printed report.

Walk at least 1 mile
Do a few yoga poses and if unfamiliar find a great video online
Enjoy a dinner: spiral sliced veggies, salad, quinoa, soup with some seaweed
Add mushrooms to your dishes and several times per week, raw Brazil nuts

Set up your sleeping area to be dark and free from electronics
Take 2 magnesium
Get to sleep if possible by 10 pm and bank up on some sleep for healing and regeneration

Your daily plan may look a little different. Perhaps you are used to fasting occasionally, and you live on a vegetarian diet for the last few years, you drink plenty of water and you are going to skip the cleanse package to prepare because you are already on your way. You may wish to use the probiotic, skin brushing and get going on iodine right away along with selenium and magnesium.

The other composition book that is your Food Diary is for you to list honestly what you ate and drank because having it in front of you will begin to show you the corresponding ways you feel with how you are eating.

The sooner you begin directly avoiding wheat, and, dairy the better as you cannot reasonably expect to heal your thyroid gland and continue eating them. Write down a plan to quit substances: cigarettes, alcohol and recreational substances. Smoking of any kind is why most people who smoke end up with hoarseness and throat problem down the road.

**Begin to notice how you spend your energy: cut out trips to the casino as it is full of cigarette smoke and EMFs. For many people that are suffering with thyroid problems start to notice when you behave compulsively** for example, shopping for clothing, and behaviors where you are always buying food and treats like running through coffee drive-through. These are draining us of positive life force energy, good for a rare treat if you want but not a regular stop.

If you are on medications take some time and review whether or not you can take any of the over the counter supplements or do a cleanse. **There are a few contraindications to using Iodine because iodine is also a blood thinner.** Please note that medications for high blood pressure, cholesterol, blood thinners, bipolar medications, and the list could keep going are something you and your doctor will have to reconcile once you finish your cleanse and you see how you feel. You would not have thick blood if you get your body and mind detoxed after a period of time the congestion will clear out. You make sure you get out and walk every single day and spend time outside in Nature; it is important that you are not just inside the car, the house, the job and school, that you get out of the box.

Many of the foods that are harming you are being consumed all the time by our families, coworkers, and everywhere, that it is like bait, you just want it! But, once you get going on learning how to prepare food, you can make cheesecakes, pies, hand dipped chocolate macaroons like I do in a fraction of the time, and they are super easy! That's why I taught a Raw Vegan GF Cheesecake class at Whole Foods this year because once people see this they can do it themselves quite easily and not feel like they have nothing delicious to eat-you do! Maybe this is something you can do as well? You could learn how to prepare these simple and delicious items that you can enjoy on your detox like raw pumpkin pie, raw apple pie and a variety of cheesecakes made with cashews or zucchini and feel good while you still enjoy some great treats!

I have seen and helped hundreds of people detox in the last 3 decades so I have good experience with the militant newbie who is never going to touch this or that and how good they feel but, they find themselves slipping up once or twice and dealing with their own inner demons getting tripped up in their feelings— **and their feelings will drive them to self sabotage, it takes strength and that's the truth; you know why? Because you are saying no to a treat!** If you get tripped up, and you have something with wheat or dairy, stay calm, and you will do better next time-acknowledge it on your Food Dairy and hit the reset and note the feelings, toilet time, nose blowing, or other symptoms on your Food Diary and get yourself back onto the Plan.

I have had clients over so many years tell me they are doing it all and nothing is working for them, or that their sneezing is just coming out of nowhere or that they **caught a cold from being around the young children at somebody's home. No way. Your body does not lie.** If you eat sweets and sugar, or grains that convert to glucose you will be sneezing the next day and you may also have bladder leakage which is commonly triggered by sugar.

After detoxification and allowing your body to reduce swelling, inflammation, congestion and mucous **you will feel the difference** and **you will observe the world quite differently.**

You notice now how all around you are others who would greatly benefit from the mental and physical clarity; how you feel now, as compared to how you felt before you detoxed.

As Arnold Ehret states in his book, **the tongue is like a sponge** and it will show you —just by learning to interpret what it is showing you. This is why after decades of understanding and hundreds of people

I can have a conversation even in the dog park and ask to see a tongue and tell a great deal.

People are loaded with waste and predictably they feel as though they have caught a cold, when their own body was gifting them with a cleansing opportunity. Just take a look next time at how much mucous you blow out, sneeze out, eliminate and is on your bowel movements and notice your urine. Arnold recommends allowing your urine to sit and then observing it. I will ask you to begin the habit of smelling your urine.

When you are full of waste, You cannot really even smell, hear or taste let alone have powerful intuitive insights about you life journey.

Many people who advertise as psychic, mediums, healers, coaches: why would I possibly rely on your insights for spiritual and intuitive direction when you are needing to detox yourself? People are full of waste. This dims your intuitive abilities, I know I have developed mine for many years and I know when they work the best, naturally they rely on my ability to use my intuition and ability to be calm and sense.

If you have undigested waste, and you consume alcohol and toxic factory farmed animals, you are not going to be able to experience sentient life force energy as well, this is just a fact. Once I began on this way of life over three decades ago I found much more clarity to quickly and easily access The Field. There is a **group that I took a course with and that I admire very much called HeartMath Institute and they teach people about the Coherent Heart Field,** highly recommended.

After you detox and heal, I guarantee that you will experience that it is far easier now to live fully present and alive and think clearly versus **using food, substances, cigarettes, alcohol, drugs, medications and people. We legitimize our sullen, drained and negative moods and lack of**

**time or ability to detox with excuses** and being too busy or that we are unable to change in an attempt to avoid doing this work of detoxification and giving yourself the gift of freedom from it and clarity.

**And, we become crystal clear how painful it is to be around most people who are entrenched in this cycle of self-infliction of emotional and physical distress and how prevalent it is all around us. How easily it can be changed!** Imagine the ways we can liberate ourselves with mental and physical clarity. This changes everything from our supermarkets to our spirituality. How we spend our time and how we listen, how we live, the work we do, the way we parent, grow, care, handle and prepare our food.

Just look at what we have today? Fruits and vegetables from the grocery store often have stickers on them and are handled numerous times, placed on conveyor belts, boxes, handled by the supermarket clerks and by the time they go home they are pretty distanced from the Earth or tree, handled as if only a product. The further we distance ourselves from food forests, growing our own food and feeling well, the more we behave mechanically and less spiritually. We become more linear and less in the way of the spiral: expansion. You see this all around you with people, dogs, animals becoming utility or things and not beings, not fully acknowledged as sentient life. **What does this have to do with your thyroid? You are constantly sensing your environment and anyone can see that the family gatherings, closeness, the ways we saw children playing outside in our neighborhoods and much of life has changed away from its organic spiral.**

We have perfect food that is nourishing from the time we are born and we partake of the breast and we are fed instantly her antibodies for us at just the right time, the nutrients and **the supply of her iodine and minerals that develops us and connects us with her microbiome, colonizes bacteria that are crucial for us to develop our intricately designed immune system**. Our palate is stimulated by sucking, and our eyes develop with the beauty of gazing into the loving eyes of our mother, we are bacteria, we are earth; that is our skin, our organs, glands, tissues, cells, bones are all made up of earth, water, air and fire: they are minerals. You cannot function without minerals.

To detox is not to become perfect or better than anybody else, it is a gift to yourself to liberate you from the freedom to feel alive and energized, and to create a life that has a higher potential to self actualize. You cannot do that if you start your day on the toilet for long periods of time, and when you are anxious and depressed, and you have multiple mucous related issues to deal with like asthma, allergies, sinus issues, pneumonia, and you are so unwell that you cause yourself (cells) to stay at that vibration through self sabotage.

To heal you and your thyroid is not difficult, it is simple. Part of why I asked you to sit quietly and observe around people around you and that while you are quiet and you observe to notice what you see with body size, energy, skin, breathing, walking, riding in carts, what they are buying and eating, and you will begin to see for yourself how all of this is most often self afflicted and then the systems we have in place cater to treating self affliction a great part of the time.

To heal your thyroid you understand now that you must give your mind and body freedom from stress and chemicals, overeating, smoking and do your walking. You have come to understand that your thyroid was repeatedly exposed to toxins in the form of radiation, heavy metals, halides like bromine, chlorine and fluoride, and toxins also found in vaccines and medications. Be patient and begin to have more quiet time to think without distraction. Prepare with your weekly shopping so that you reduce your need to go run out and get food.

Prepare by obtaining an HTMA, Hair Tissue Mineral Analysis written report done just for you so that you can see what you need to focus on and replenish; this will save a lot of time and grief as well as money wondering what supplements to get just for you! You can find the HTMA link on my website at www.naturallywithkaren.com.

In **Professor Arnold Ehret's Mucusless Diet Healing System-Scientific Method Eating Your Way to Health**, which can be found for free online through truthseekerz, you can read about how fasting cures just about everything, many other people had centers and retreats where you could go and obtain supervised fasting.

It is interesting to me that the same message with a different twist by a different proclaimer, artist or writer, is being repeated and stated over and over to those **who have never heard it**: you are what you eat and if you eat fruits and starch-less vegetables and observe your tongue, your body, urine and bowel movements you will see for yourself that as many a new guru appears touting that we have no mystery disease, it is the same message just a different messenger. Arnold published The Mucusless Diet Healing System in 1953 and he had terrific results but many also came before him and a great many after him. We are all saying the same thing: You are your own physician and you know yourself enough to heal yourself. 99% of the time I do not need intervention: not a colonoscopy, not a mammogram, not vaccines, not X-rays, Not MRI, Not CT Scans, Not medications, Not most surgeries, none of it, except for wounds, burns, accidents that need trauma care.

We are requiring more from the doctor today than ever before!

Everywhere I look **people are disabling themselves by becoming starch stiff and inflexible,** mentally and physically and **it is no mystery to me why their thyroid and my own became imbalanced.** Our lack of ease collectively as people is centered in the throat right now due to our collective pain. **Our pain is that we are choking, we are not able to speak out and we are gasping for real life again, but too few of us** remember what that even is, and have despairing thoughts or have given up on ever reaching natural life again, so we continue coping and in our despair we eat more, recreationally, and we stuff ourselves with products that are created to cause us to sink into food coma. Cheap products like cake snacks, and 12 packs of soft drinks, diet drinks, muffins, cookies, and the same stuff is being sold at nearly every coffee shop, how boring and toxic!

We have new forms of communication today, on our phones, through our computer, and in many ways, long past the fax now, we can send data and information instantly. This is what we do with energy and, it has been tested! We can think of someone and we can send them healing energy on the spot, it works! But what about what is coming up ahead now?

Radio active is communication becoming ready. Your thyroid gland sits directly in front on your neck, and it is your sensor, your ability to speak your true self, be heard and have a voice.

What is sustainable? It means that not only my generation at age 56, but future generations are thought of equally and have a place to live on Earth.

I can speak with any other person over the age of 45 and they realize that we cannot sustain the directions we are going with any reasonable form of sanity. We cannot keep producing drugs in response to maladies of mind and heart that now manifest in the body. We cannot keep using plastics that contain exogenous estrogens and which affect your progesterone levels and cause so many hormonal issues as well as landfill issues and issues at sea.

I realize, I have given you a lot of information. I kept it simple and in plain English and easy to understand. I have given you other books that will greatly compliment your journey should you be interested as well as tidbits that will provoke thought, including increasing awareness about sustainability.

I could have written about 10 pages in a manual which had just basic detox, dietary, lifestyle pieces of awareness relative to our thyroid gland, thyroid imbalance, thyroid disease, exposures, environment, minerals, halides, but I made this into a way of life: a journey for you.

What I do and offer here in this book is entirely different from appearing at a doctor's office and asking somebody else to do it for you. **It's not a gamut of testing to prove or disprove a diagnosis code,** nor is this way all about taking just one pill, or one fix.

This book is about detoxification, healing, and a way of life: building into a sustainable awareness, so we can all continue living a good life, something I have often throughout this book referred to as becoming your own physician.

Know thyself and heal thyself: self love alongside being willing and able to truly procure self discipline to set in place daily habits is essential. You have choices, you can do it all yourself just using this book and greatly benefit from it, and, you can also have somebody do consults with you. Some people hire others to prepare their meals, make their juices, and other prepare their weekly shopping ahead of time, order HTMA and get going on their supplements.

Start by reading through the book, then, doing the first three easy aspects of pre-detox: get your probiotic and put it into your refrigerator, get a skin brush and hang it where you will see it and use it. And, get some clay or DE and set up your plan.

Get to sleep a bit earlier and recharge each night that you are able. Get your supplements together and plan out how you will get walking in Nature if possible-different from a treadmill. Release tension, absorb sunlight, and breathe outdoors-deeply into your belly and come out of upper chest breathing and fully oxygenate your cells. Give yourself some quiet time to set up a plan for yourself, I realize everything shared in this book may not feel like a great fit for everyone, so I made sure to include many of the aspects of healing your thyroid that I would often relate with clients in consultation. An aspect of the book may not be at your comfort level right now and yet it may be at another time.

You can decrease inflammation in your thyroid gland, and, have real tools that will reduce cysts, nodules and help you to restore health in your thyroid gland by detoxing, knowing which foods are causing your direct harm, congesting your body and producing more cysts like wheat and cheese.

Begin to get familiar with seaweeds: put them in soups, salads or other ways. By consuming  foods with iodine it will help you to detox your organs. Become educated about the truth about taking synthetic thyroid hormone-holding an expectation that it will heal you may not be realistic; you have other options, perhaps, bioidentical hormone replacement therapy "BHRT."

It is entirely realistic to expect your body to be able to detox and for you to heal your own thyroid or, shrink thyroid nodule, I believe it is. Can you begin to calm your autoimmune issues-yes you can!  Do not expect to hear sovereign choices for healing yourself in the mainstream today, it won't happen yet, but it will! Thyroid pain is big business and, thyroid medication is likely still one of the most common "medication" being sold today. With fast food, fast life, we also want fast healing and, it doesn't work that way. And, the more realistic and sustainable we become, the fewer problems with drugs in our societies we will have, because we genuinely become a model worthy of imitation.

I know you can do this and you can pick and choose what you want to do and when you do it, review it with your doctor, or health coach and do what feels right for you!

Once we know, then we must do better!

Most of us would not spray toxic pesticides around our young children, nor, ourselves, we would do not want to eat toxic food, nor drink contaminated water. None of us want to eat animal products which contain growth hormones, antibiotics and other chemicals which are in the immunizations given to the animals. Fragranced and artificial body and hair care products are also polluting our glands and organs. It is offensive to walk by some folks outside on trails or in shopping areas who have a great deal of fragrance from head to toe.

**We are missing iodine, our mothers are missing iodine and together with exposures to far too many halogens:** chemicals in our drinking, tooth brushing, bathing, and showering water, as well as preparing our foods in this water, we are exposing ourselves far too often to chlorine, fluoride and perhaps other heavy metals and contaminants that are directly affecting our thyroid gland.

I discussed ways that we can reduce exposures and why we would want to and the negative effects to our skin's mantle. People are just learning now that they should eliminate using **sunscreen as it is harmful in reducing our ability to make secosteriod hormone D also known as vitamin D from sunlight.** If we are toxic and congested from ingesting wheat, dairy and factory farmed meats, chances are our skin will not assimilate nor eliminate well and could cause it to have lesions on the skin that could become cancerous under the right conditions.

### Ozone Therapy

Ozone therapy is done to heal the thyroid gland and restore balance. Dr. Brownstein, M.D., has spoken about this and you can contact their office for more information. In the event you do not know about this, you can look into it since I do to do it but wanted to make sure you are aware of it and perhaps it may work for you.

### Make it Happen!

While many people will set their mind and accomplish their plan and they do it, they are now past the issue of detox and heal their thyroid and onto life betterment and improvement by way of their intention and self discipline, other people will buy a book and never sit down and read it. We are either doers or we are not. I hope you are a doer and that you not only read through this book and enjoy it, but that it opens your mind and that you, heal yourself. You always had that ability, the same way you could many things in life, I believe in you! Healthier, happier people mean a safer, better world for us all, and certainly most people would agree a world with less drugs, prescribed and, on the streets.

However, many people exclusively look for some treatment and many for very good reason, pain is no fun! I would be absolutely rich today if I just sold some special spray, cream, pill or something that promises the moon and back, but I peddle my decades of gathering experience and healing myself as well as guiding many others.

I know that people often stop short of completing their goals and I know a thing or two about self sabotage. For this reason, there is snake oil on every corner and great people selling it every day. In fact, it gives us a bad name when young people sell all the MLM products with all their promises or somebody promises that their smoothies will cure anything. Again, it is a way of life that optimizes your quality of life and what you experience; what you put in is what you get out of it. There are no shortcuts.

Ninety percent of people lack iodine, and most doctors will scare you away from it. People became congested and their thyroid gland became inflamed and slow. Nobody noticed just like when I was young as a girl with all the glaring signs of low blood pressure, low body temperature, breech birth, photophobia, and all the rest, developmentally, and more, and I did not notice with my son that he became Myxedemic after nearly dying at the hospital at 6 days of age, and rebalanced, and then a big move which related in a lot of stress, then puberty hit and he again suffered by way of a poor diet after coming to Minnesota and the onset of puberty hormones. Our poor children are being labeled with ODD when they are so low on energy reserves that they finally cannot stand the incessant anxiety, racing mind and heart and panic that sets in when the sluggish thyroid is overtaxes and becomes a hyperthyroid and has runaway symptoms that produce rabid irritability, moods, insomnia that is almost untreatable at times, and doctors send them home with sleeping medications including Ambien and they nearly lose their minds, it costs them relationships and goals in life because we fail them with setting standards as the same thing is happening with society it too is runaway with false standards and unrealistic role models poised as celebrities that spew negative and self deprecating models of behavior. Where are we to stop it? We are being choked from telling the truth that we know to be true. We, must be the change.

### Dr. Jeckyl & Mr. Hyde

If you detox and I realize nearly everyone reading this will say, but how do I get off wheat it is everywhere? I know, and, so is thyroid imbalance although it is not diagnosed, it's there! If you detox and you go back to eating and living as you did before, it will not be fun, your body will remind you in unpleasant ways that it wants to be fed. I am reminded of a dog I saw today at the dog park who kept begging for a piece of meat, as the man was was munching on a cheeseburger and the dog beginning desperately for a piece of it was denied..I said to the man as kindly as possible, **"I bet your** companion there would like some meat." **The man just looked at me; almost puzzled.** The dog knows what he needs and the dog lays down when it gets dark unless he lives in a home full of loud blaring noise and TVs and such then it is awfully uncomfortable for the dog who would lay down once it gets dark, it's innate in the animal for self protection when it got dark and for health. You too have to know better and do better, even if it feel odd at first, find what you can do and allow yourself to feel good about it.

You may know the story of Dr. Jekyll and Mr. Hyde-of how one man ended up with a split personality? This is reality for people who detoxify and heal, then binge on wheat cookies, and "*fill up*" again.

Our food industry has set up programs within the population that repeat the same language: rewards and "*treats.*" We are very treat driven, and after we work, or make some sort of sacrifice of our time and energy, we "treat" ourselves and gift ourselves with oral gratification, even when we are not hungry. Eating is enjoyable and we reward ourselves with eating what we like and what tastes good. Freud has much to say about oral gratification and our missing our mother.

If you detox and eat clean and then, occasionally, veer from eating clean, no big deal; but **detoxify and gain your thyroid function and health back, and then, go back to stuffing, wheat, and lots of chemicals and you too will feel as if you look like Hyde!**

When people have substantial thyroid imbalance they want to *hide*, and **isolate** and **recluse** isn't this what is happening today? There are always clues in many of our old stories! I bet you're laughing right now because it's true!

Historically, we had asylums and hospitals that people were placed into and they were horrific! Women were commonly put in their place and if they were outspoken or too powerful like Frances Farmer, and others they suffered with lobotomy or insane asylums or worse! Part of why we call one of most common surgeries a hysterectomy is due to the hysterical uterus effect that speaks of women as being hysterical. Over 9 million of us died during the witchcraft trials and I have heard it had to do with bacteria in the rye and of course monopoly.

Even in today's world, I met with a doctor recently in Duluth, MN that is not my doctor but to help somebody and to partner in the health of another person we both see. **The medical profession by and large will not acknowledge that there are many mental and emotional issues that people with thyroid imbalance face and suffer from?** Can you imagine how many people could have been helped? Even a handful of modern psychiatrists are waking up in the last decade to removing drugs from their practices.

I have been relating about reversing cancer since the 1980s to anything you suffer from most of the time, it is that easy! I have even given talks that were entirely FREE at local establishments and people hesitate to believe it?

I wrote this book as well because many people with thyroid issues would love to know what to do for themselves and they have more than one diagnosis, many of my clients has several at time that were all interconnected around thyroid as a basis or root cause.

In recent times, many people who suffered emotionally and mentally were not truly helped but were placed into mental health hospitals, specialty centers because we did not know? If I can know, how come the bulk of doctors today in clinics and hospitals including many endocrinologists do not know? An Endocrinologist is a hormone specialist and I have never heard of one that recommends detoxification and mineral balancing, including the element iodine! And, if you are a Doctor or Endocrinologist and you do, please contact me with an email I would love to hear from you.

In order to communicate our truth and our nature—and this is truly what our thyroid gland is teaching us at this time in life we need to take a look at, and strengthen our way of life.

Far too many children are diagnosed as Oppositional Defiant, impulsive, it is way too common to be diagnosed as ADHD, and so many other ways we diagnose and drug children today in this attempt to maintain our sanity in a world begging for change-we cannot ignore our thyroid! If we do, we have run our vehicles too far into the ground with the check engine light blaring a red beacon at us that is now too loud to ignore!

We have everything we need to resurrect life with health so why not look at it? We make many of the drugs found on the streets illegal, yet we allow foods that are without a doubt, drugs that are making people sick every single day with disease codes that never end.

More drugs, more advertisements with promises, more frustrated parents, and yet the answers are right before us, except that the drugs are some of the most addicting on the planet! Doctors and meds are paid for through our insurance company so nothing comes out of our pocket and, we are unfamiliar with consulting.

People who suffer with thyroid imbalance are very intelligent they have had to learn how to maneuver in life with feeling more tired and worn out and perhaps at the same time, have high copper levels and be very intense, they often feel as if they are just hard wired to be this way, but pleasantly surprised when they do an HTMA and find out that we can begin to bring down that copper high intensity personality with zinc.

We need Elders who can be part of a Council that is collaborative, and truly able to agree to disagree and find consensus for the betterment of all. People who are not on substances of any kind and are clean of mind and heart. People who are driven towards restoring humanity and people healing in some of these ways and growing food together in food forests.

We have to rethink our reward and punishment language and redirect our many habits.

## Becoming Anointed

Our glands, including our thyroid gland all communicate. Our pituitary gland, pineal gland, thyroid, thymus, adrenals, pancreas, and sex organs. Cholesterol makes many of our hormones and the hormones are circulated throughout the body with glands and made and also used by our organs.

For us to "vibrate" is music! This energetic vibration has everything to do with the function of our glands and thus our nutrition, energy, lifestyles, and environmental exposures, minerals, enzymes and rest will enhance or disrupt this energy.

To be anointed is very *similar* to being luminous and experiencing not just an actualized life, but one of integrity, honesty and one where you begin to sense beyond the mechanical level. You no longer see through the lens of just treating your parts, or in the same way, eating as just getting energy, but you vibrate in accordance with Nature. You begin to sense all beings with respect. You need your glands to be free of cysts, nodules, calcification and parasites.

In some of our oldest books, and, The Bible, it speaks to our being "anointed". There are images that we can find when we search out the meaning-what does it means-to be, anointed? What I have found most commonly, is an image where you see somebody with some sort of an oil being placed on the top of their head. Other images show a horn that is used to contain the special oil for this purpose and then in passages or images refers to a direct connection to God; to any expression of God, our spirituality or, our religion. There are most definitely missing pieces that we seek, and long for to connect with The Field, the energy matrix that is essentially, plasma.

Our pineal gland rests just under where the infants "soft spot," or "fontanelle," is, just inches below this area, which takes an infant about a year to close up and secure after birth-for the cranium to fully mature. For this reason, we keep the head covered which is the crown, out in public amongst the many energies or the public until after this time, and we are protective of this area. This is part of ripening your sacred glands and being able to protect yourself, and develop your inner sight and wisdom. Many of our habits today, are harmful like people bringing young babies out and among loud noises, at concerts, while their fontanelle is still open to the world and their glands are still developing. For example, our coating on our nervous system; our myelin sheath is developing for approximately two years after we are born. If we are mineral deficient we begin life in a state of poverty.

Our current ways of life have been broken for hundreds of years and then are progressively more and more broken: the result produced is people who are hormonally deranged, heavily medicated, and they are walking science experiments. The misery some of the parents go through when their children are assaulted by a system such as this one causes not only fatigue, and exhaustion, but it renders us separated from the whole (tribe), and traumatized.

There is talk of the building of facilities as our young adults will have shortened lifespans due the multigenerational mineral deficits, glandular imbalances and the effects of consuming genetically modified organisms for food. The disconnection of sending children to school younger and younger is yet another 'study' that reinforces separation of child from mother and the home and hearth from humanity as we are choked into becoming utility singularly and exclusively serving the machine.

At one time people ate real food, they grew it and they needed relatively little compared to the thousands of pounds consumed by just one individual in today's world, very little of it nutrient or mineral dense due to our depleted soils. Our problems are not about tired soils, they are about failing to become sustainable with agriculture as a community and not singularly the glut of a corporation; again, mechanical compared to organic.

Our glands are already under assault with so many of the ways we live today, with higher numbers of vaccinations, chemicals in the environment, and mothers who are deficient in minerals so necessary to fund their energy and gift to their babies. **They and their children end up with thyroid imbalance because to host a child internally requires the gift of their minerals and if they themselves do not have enough the child is born without enough as well** and so this is why children are as unwell as they are and are producing many of the behaviors that we call ADHD, ODD and other names today. The multigenerational aspects of thyroid disease should now be far more simple to understand, do you see?

**If mother, grandmother and great grandmother were all mineral deficient than we have progressively diminished our family** and then, we add the denatured commercial supermarket foods of today. Wheat is very inexpensive, it is in everything, chicken nuggets, to breaded coatings on fish, pancakes, waffles, muffins, toast, sandwiches, and we suffer by inflaming our internal organs, developing rashes, irritating our gut and, then **we medicate**.

Many of the medications contain sodium salts which produce problems because now your potassium or other minerals levels are very off balanced and the both suffers from internal swelling. This could also cause brain swelling which also can arise from commercially sprayed berries and foods sold at commercial grocery stores which contain bromide and sodium salts. Swelling in the brain can compromise your upper glands: pituitary and pineal.

You need your pineal gland to sleep well, to make DMT and many other functions that also co-relate with your pituitary gland which makes part of the hormones necessary for your thyroid. In fact, the most common testing done by doctors today is to check your TSH and compare your numbers on a range as we discussed much earlier in the book. If your pituitary gland is not working well then your hormones will be compromised and your thyroid gland will also begin to become imbalanced. Our glands do not just become imbalanced for no reason at all. They become off balance due to many reasons. One is that are living within a sea of signals electronically that disrupt our brain. Enough research has been done to prove that not only do cell phones disrupt thyroid hormones, but they do quite a bit more.

# CHAPTER THIRTEEN - PREVENTION

We know that radiation could be minimized, especially in our lifestyle and our home, work, and, school environments. We do not need as many X-rays and CT Scans, children carrying cell phones, tablets and gaming systems. Something I really appreciated about Waldorf School is that they wait on the technology and books until at least after age 7, it is not rushed as it is in the mainstream world.

By now, we know that we need iodine in our diet as well as perhaps as a supplement. We need to evaluate our minerals and toxic exposures so that we can prevent instead of deal with emergencies that could be prevented. Your thyroid gland needs iodine, your thyroid hormones in part are made of iodine, but you also need iodine to for your ovaries, breast, prostate, eyes, brain, cerebrospinal fluid, salivary glands, and, according to Jorge Flechas, M.D., a "definite increase in the incidence of breast cancer, stomach cancer, ovarian cancer and thyroid cancer with the presence of iodine deficiency."

Iodine significantly reduces cancer rates, detoxifies your internal organs, thins the blood and is very healing for every cell of the body. Because of bromine in all of our foods and products it blocks our ability to use iodine. Radioactive iodine also displaces our iodine. According to Dr. Brownstein, M.D., patients cannot find iodine knowledgeable healthcare practitioners. I know every time I have gone into the natural foods store people are only aware of kelp tablets, the very small dosage of transdermal iodine and much like the calcium and protein programs the iodine discomfort is very real. Kelp tablets and bleached Japanese seaweed products will not render a therapeutic dose of iodine. I personally take 50 and have taken more and done quite well on it for quite some time.

People can take iodine as soon as they are ready provided that they review what medications they are on meaning many of them have sodium salts in their makeup which interfere with people's potassium levels and other minerals. Children can often take iodine and so can adults and elders with great benefit.

Once you are on your path and well established and healing is well underway, and you will know because of the way you swallow, your feel, your energy, your skin, your bowel movement, your urine, your tongue, your eyes, and people will be commenting on how amazing you look! Remember, to take your (BBTs), temperature periodically, These ways I have related in this book will help you to recognize when you are not in balance. You are aware that a venous blood sample likely may not be definitive to bring your awareness to doing what you need to do for yourself: detox & heal.

We can begin to prevent much of what we are experiencing. There were long years when the body was giving warnings, but we were not given the instructions on how to care for ourselves nor truly listen to the glaring warnings in our childhood days. The wheat rashes on our skin, the hyper pigmentation that we just dismissed, the skin tags, the eczema, asthma, allergies, sleep apnea (congestive), and the alarming rate of esophageal cancers and gut disorders. Our thyroid gland is just one part of our cells that make up you. If you rely on somebody else to **exclusively** check and treat you, you may wait too long. This book is specifically to detox and heal yourself but there is a lot you can do to improve your health.

I also respect doctors for their knowledge and abilities and I realize that they have limitations imposed upon them-they have amazing insights as well, it would be great to see more for people with prevention earlier with children.

Prevention includes keeping a healthy gut and diet, as well as lifestyle. Minimizing exposure to harmful EMFs and radiation. That equates to reducing the number of X-rays, CT scans, and talking with children on road trips instead of placing our children in front of screens as we travel on road trips. It means talking with them about real life, and about knowing themselves.

Thyroid gland issues almost always have some aspects of not being able to speak our truth, or feel heard and so we need better communication styles and practices with each other and we need to overcome the scarcity and lack programs that we all deal with today, whether it is money, popularity for our teens, acceptance, we have no shortage of them and we can overcome them, each of us individually and empower ourselves again through right living and simplifying down, reducing, recycling are not just buzz words. I live simple and I love it!

We need to know our human body again. I mean, that most often my clients rarely ever touched their neck and throat and did not know they have lumpy bumpy cysts all over is telling. Teach children about their glands earlier on and how to take care of them and feed their cells. Let's educate for heath and not mediocrity, like sharing with people as to why we feed our cells and about why we need minerals-let's have real conversations about why we allow the food industry that we do.

Many people feel that vaccines are absolutely necessary and this book is not to debate the use of vaccines it is to speak to the toxic ingredients which have been and continue to be present in the vaccines themselves like aluminum and mercury as well as others.

We need preparation and education that is better suited to cause people to begin experiencing more meaningful and successful lives so that we do not despair so often and feel **humiliated** about some of the choices we must make to continue our existence economically and strategically to keep in accordance with all the modern ways, rules and regulations that often do not serve humanity but enforce and reduce.

Whether you are a doctor, police officer, teacher, mother, grandparent, or a teenager reading this book, I am with you, you are part of the human family and thyroid issues are affecting everybody today and we can do something about it.

**We, are off balance and we all want balance again even if we do not want to make changes like I suggest in this book.** This book is my passion.

Let's avoid black and white thinking: I'm not a "tree hugger," I am somebody who truly cares and who gathered from many resources for long decades and I hold out hope for humanity for a World Family.

I have seen a lot, interviewed people while working in Family Law, in the Courts, The District Attorney and law firms, as well as consultations now for nearly 15 years.

**This book is a seed-one that I have planted with heart,** it took me years to clearly express what I have to share with you and I believe it wholeheartedly, I live it. It healed me several times and I am a survivor of thyroid in my family which was hit very hard by thyroid issues, I know them now, inside and out now. I am somebody who had to be absolutely sure that I felt and stand by what I say here, and, I live it.

You prevent by knowing what to look for and having the tools. Filtering your water, knowing about your shower water, redirecting your thoughts into positive ways, and engaging with your Mind Body Medicine aspects of thyroid imbalance which are in part, **humiliation.**

Taking some quiet time and truly introspecting within yourself and gaining clarity about you, your journey and your health and life.

You got this! And, I'm with you!

# CHAPTER FOURTEEN - MY STORY

Our stories are medicine. People can relate many of their own experiences with a story, and stories are shared; many people learn and benefit from them. It is my hope that people who read this story of mine about myself and my son that it will help to correct or prevent negative experiences and illness from happening. Thyroid symptoms made themselves known from birth for both myself and my son. I reversed my symptoms of thyroid imbalance and you can too.

The difference between detox and heal your thyroid and just using one synthetic thyroid hormone, or, ignoring, or covering up the symptoms, is the difference between having a good life and a life of pain: physically, emotionally, mentally, and spiritually. Thyroid imbalances can cause so many problems on each of these levels. Thyroid-related anxiety is often is what will drive people to alcohol and drug addiction. Thyroid imbalance and iodine deficiency produce many of our learning disabilities and throughout the years what was called "mental retardation." Suicides are a major concern today that would be far less of a worry if we reduced the anxiety and depression, that people encounter when needing a detox so that they can regenerate their health. Iodine is needed for every cell in the body and most people can begin eating seaweeds that I mention in the book, and most people can begin taking a 12.5 mg iodine/iodide supplement like Iodoral in addition to a detox and find tremendous benefit! Throughout many decades I observed that many of our diseases today are treated, but not truly healed. Detoxification, diet, iodine, food based vitamin C, and minerals, for rebalancing thyroid imbalances are not commonly discussed with people by their doctors, nor are many health care practitioners available for people who have this knowledge to steer them in the direction of knowledge of self and, self healing. This book breaks down each category for you to understand the how, where, when and why so that you can empower yourself, heal yourself and know how easy it is! Making us all strong and healthy is a foundation to building unity and cooperation.

I began to understand a little at a time after my son nearly died at six days of age as I was unable to breast feed; I lacked mammary gland tissue. That caused many other events to happen which changed our lives. I spent years to understand what was happening; I was tested a few times and found that if I cared about myself and my family, as well as my clients I have to keep searching - I have to find the truth. Then, I had to put together a plan and stick to it and heal myself.

What motivated me? Being live to raise my son as a solo parent on our own-I wanted to be here for him. I know now that I was so toxic for a period of time, that when clients came to me years later to relate that they felt almost insane, I was never arrogant enough to say I knew what they were going through, but I said, I believe I may be able to understand what that may feel like. Thyroid imbalances, especially with adrenal exhaustion, and a need to detox are why we have so many migraines, cancer, Crohn's Disease, Fibromyalgia, and other problems that could be prevented. I believe the brain tumors are in part caused by the fibrin based issues generated by thyroid imbalance. Iodine helps clear cysts, nodules and some tumors because it is detoxifying and thins the blood. **Most of us are deficient in iodine and we consume foods that further congest the body causing it to make and hold onto more cysts.**

**Some folks suggest that likely 90% of people in the Great Lakes Regions have thyroid issues.** The most difficult aspect of what I do is to bring this awareness and so I decided to write this book.

I was born **breech**, feet first and a tad low in **birthweight** at about 6 pounds, with green eyes, at a Kaiser Hospital in San Francisco, California as my parents were residing in Cupertino, CA. My mother relates that the doctors at Kaiser told her that my eyes were noted as being **light sensitive (Photophobia).**

I would have never made the connections that breech birth, low birthweight, photophobia, left handedness, and many of the other things I experienced in my life had anything to do with thyroid imbalance, but they do. I have read about them in several books about thyroid written by doctors.

In elementary school at Henry S. Hammer school in San Jose, I naturally gravitated to writing with my left hand and was quickly identified as a **left hander.** That was not accepted, even in California at that time around 1966. The teacher forced a few students to write with their right hand so I had a bit of practice and development with my right hand. My mother came in to speak with the teacher and advocated for me telling the teacher that I was to write with what hand I felt inclined. I am aware that in other parts of the country people had a hand tied behind their back, or were hit with a ruler! Much as in the same way, in my early grades girls were not allowed to wear pants.

Several times I was taken to the doctor for an annual physical exam perhaps for back to school as it was something that schools were asking parents to do and some were requiring. I know for sure that my family was not too fond of "*doctoring*." During your physical exam several predictable things happen. Blood pressure, temperature, sticking your tongue out, and checking your reflexes, at least back then. I, always had **low body temperature** and **low blood pressure**. Additionally, I had a **poor ankle reflex** when they hit you softly with that plexor on key points to check your reflexes and uses a score between 0-4, mine did not move at all; **zero means that your electricity is not flowing well** and four means that you are overreactive. Does this make sense? If your electricity is not flowing because your thyroid has been slowed there will be a delay in your reflexes. To this day I am extremely light sensitive and just cannot look towards the sun, it is called "**Photophobia**." Common to people who experienced radiation exposures, we have some structural issues, often scoliosis or can have a **coccyx which protrudes** a bit which I picked up on more so later in life in yoga that I found it difficult to do some of the floor poses and made that connection: we view ourselves as just "normal," throughout our lives. In utero exposure to **radioactive iodine occupies the thyroid** and fills the spaces that would normally have iodine. The thyroid gland begins to slow and the person slows in the same way, until they have gone too long without help.

Who would I have been and how would I have chosen to live my life without having been poisoned by ionizing radiation and mercury? How many thousands of people could ask themselves this question and how many of our relatives left prematurely from goiters, and lymphocytic issues that are often related to radiation exposures. Many of them our men who served in the military for this country.

We visit our doctors expecting to receive care and knowledge of what is happening in the world in terms of our health and we give our trust to them to let us know as they are the standard of care for us yet, I have been disappointed and so have many others by the regulated care that is a part of the standardized curriculum of the AMA.

Every one of us has been in a flimsy gown in a cold room on a table waiting for the doctor feeling disempowered and vulnerable, feeling **humiliated** and reduced. It almost feels like the way it is set up is something close to the cattle of today and how they must feel in factory farming. How many people have waited to hear what they have?

About the age of 12, I went to the dentist and, he indicated that I had 23 spot **cavities**. The lucky Dentist who benefited from my father's insurance plan, filled the entire tooth with amalgam mercury fillings which I had in my mouth until about 2004/2005 when I sought to get them removed.

They came out thanks to a local dentist, Dr. Ludwig, at Cloquet Dental, and, he was the only dentist after seeing several in California before arriving to Minnesota in 2002 when I tried to get them taken out to no avail even with high priced spa dentists, they gave up on me, but Dr. Ludwig was able to use the numbing agent just right so that I was able to sit and relax to the degree I was able while enduring the work to remove them on numerous sessions.

Having **old metallic fillings and crowns including a variety of metals** in your mouth combined   with bacteria produce internal infections which also produce anxiety, stress and stress and your thyroid gland do not work.

I can remember the many trips I made to the local dentist's office for dental work, my little body stressed and frozen with fear at times. He used nitrous oxide each time for the lengthy visits drilling and filling each tooth all the way down. As you might imagine or you may know yourself from experiences, I was pretty terrorized by the experience and to this day suffer from some dental anxiety, he was less than patient and kind.

As a young girl I felt really vulnerable on the nitrous and out of my mind such that now the thought of the mask and that smell coming down towards my face produces a sick feeling-more **humiliation**.

I remember the positive feedback from teachers like Mrs. Hunt in first grade about my exceptional reading and communication skills. Yet, after the extensive dental work, **I became almost learning disabled, way down to below average.** I would try so hard to read a book but my comprehension was just way off; I would have to repeat the page over and over and I just could not get concepts as they were introduced. In third grade and on I realized I was **very tall,** especially compared to my classmates and I now know that thyroid gland imbalances produce **giantism** as well as **dwarfism** it causes developmental issues structurally and otherwise.

Many years ago I read the book, Thyroid Mind Power, by Dr. Shames, I realized that there were many more symptoms that I had been experiencing that were related to my thyroid-especially mental and emotional. Reading or better yet, hearing somebody else's story is the largest part of medicine. **We always provided medicine as Elders**. I am sharing a story about what you need to pick up on and learn about: **Radioactive damages done to our thyroid which continue to be used amongst our people, even in Europe recently.**

I was affected in utero by radiation, toxic heavy metals in the form of dentistry and vaccines. I was affected by a food industry that plaques and plagues people with **grain**, or wheat that is specifically **designed** and **bred** to produce beneficial crops for the farmer and yield profits but is a grain selected for other purposes. I drank city water that was full of halogens like chlorine and fluoride and as time has gone by it is increasingly full of disclosed and undisclosed contaminants that mutate our genes.

You may be saying to yourself much like I would, that it is very likely—that doctors did not know what they know today. That they did not realize a low body temperature, and all of the other signs evidenced a slow, or hypothyroidism. Then why did the **PKU heel stick officially arrive in 1963** which checked for hypothyroidism? I began to closely look at the many ways I was "checked," and nothing really ever came from it-if somebody had a temperature it was brought down but in the old ways it was our own internal fire to heat up the body and help to heal it.

From the time of the Cold War we have been building an artificial intelligence, increased communications through radio frequency and constructed The Net. The **radio active** iodine has generated a problem for humanity, but has been a benefit for technology and engineering. What I am saying is there has been significant change since 1942 that affects each one of us in profound ways and, our thyroid gland. We have more anxiety with technology that relies upon signals and electromagnetic waves. It drives us to want to be inside our homes more as if to shelter us from the sea of signals. Technology definitely amplifies anxiety.

Remembering how excited I was to have breasts and my own period, I kept waiting for that late development to come, however, all my friends got theirs before me. My sexual development was much later.

I kept hoping that I would get my "period" with the other girls around age 12, 13, 14, but mine came at **16 years of age and my breasts never did develop**. I was thoroughly embarrassed that I remained in a AA or an A cup and I was told, not to worry that when I had a baby it would all be different and they would fill out-nope. I thoroughly love my body now and my small breasts but not having enough minerals, and **being exposed to radiation and toxic heavy metals changed me in many ways, some that are scientifically studied and others that are not**.

In high school I remember how fun it seemed to have a nickname, a few called me **"turtle."** I did not put that together at that time or being slowed, I did not pay that much attention to it. As I wrote this book, I had a small silver and green metallic turtle by me, reminding me of how, I, detoxed and healed my thyroid and thus, my life. I never graduated high school and I only hoped to be a mother and a wife for most of my life. I just wanted a simple life, I love making food and sharing it. I longed to be a mother and a great one. I was quite sure I was challenged and although people enjoyed books I just could not get past the first page or two.

Again, it should have been obvious that I was failing my classes and not attending except for Psychology where I did really well. For a time after high school my parents had moved to Citrus Heights, CA and then on to Minnesota to buy land and become more "safe," I found it difficult to be organized and I knew something was not right, but I couldn't get enough brain power going to organize my thoughts enough to figure out what it was that was plaguing me.

I gained weight, I felt sleepy most of the time: tired, **sluggish**, **over-weight**, and my once beautiful hair became coarse, thinner and it became curly.

With each monthly cycle, I experienced painful PMS, cramps, and clots. I remember having a sharp pain on one of my ovaries and being told I needed to visit a gynecologist. At that time, during the checkup, the gynecologist explained about phantom cysts on the ovaries-they were a bit painful. So, I had a cyst or cysts on my ovaries and I was told they would just come and go. Today, with young women plagued by lots of cysts and for simple and obvious reasons they are called POLY cystic ovarian syndrome.

"Copperheads," seem to be increasing in numbers today. I believe that my mother was likely "**high copper**" while she was pregnant with me. Trace elements like copper and others are affected by radiation, food, vaccines, dental work, water pipes and more. Beginning in high school and even more so in my 20s and 30s many people commented on the copper streaks in my hair and often made comments about gold spots in my eyes when I was in the sunlight it was especially noticeable.

Having a copper imbalance will create a lot of problems; any mineral or trace element imbalance will. Being a high copper being or "copperhead," caused me to become officially diagnosed at one time with **Gilbert's Syndrome (high bilirubin)**. I was jaundiced and the sclera of my eyes (the white part) was extremely yellow and all the tests for Hepatitis at that time, were positive. My bilirubin was quite high and, I was told by doctors that my children had a 50% chance of also having Gilbert's Disease or Gilbert's Syndrome as it is called, either way.

**I no longer have any trace of Gilbert's Syndrome, elevated bilirubin because it is cured**.

Over the years between the ages of 21 and 30, I have had pap smears and been told I had cervical dysplasia and been through a few gynecological procedures that I am aware now, could have been entirely avoided with detoxification, mineral restoration and balance and healing through diet and way of life. I now see the obvious.

Around 1993 I was told I would never have a child after trying to conceive to no avail for many months and I scheduled a meeting with an **Infertility** Specialist Doctor, Jose Bolanos, MD. At that meeting, I was told that I had **endometriosis** and likely would not be able to become pregnant. I set out to make a plan and reversed that situation as well. The benefit of living close to the ocean was that I healed more quickly absorbing iodine. Negative ions are received from the ocean or moving water. Walking on the sand barefoot is very restorative, which would seem really '*hocus pocus*' to some people, but our integumentary system is receiving as bioavailable molecular iodine through the soles of the feet. From ages 22 to 42 I lived in the Santa Cruz Mountains and after my son was born, closer than a block to the ocean. My son and I lived in an incredibly beautiful place with beautiful nature, weather and very friendly people who all were very content living in Santa Cruz. We had great things to do, and plenty of open minded people to have meaningful conversations with at local cafes and music shows. After we moved to Minnesota due to cost of living as Santa Cruz is quite costly and many people were displaced particularly after the dot.com it was sad it was a relocation I felt I had to make but did not want to make at that time and for many years.

I conceived months later after seeing the evidence of my cleansing and detox through my monthly cycle and ended up having a **miscarriage** at 9 weeks due to a **blighted ovum**-an egg that never keeps dividing. Anybody going through a miscarriage I feel for you! What a tough time to go through! A lot of pain emotionally. I can easily remember the feelings I had, observing every stroller that goes by especially one time sitting at Los Gatos Coffee Roasting Company as I did then; wondering if that will ever be me with a baby! Following a D&C I conceived again fairly soon. My due date was August 1995.

Being pregnant was amazing, I loved every minute of it!

I was really excited about home birth, not doing the vaccines, and certainly not doing "formula!" I consulted and retained a midwife, "Rain," of Morgan Hill, to assist with a water/home birth. We bought the birth kit, and, as far as a tub to give birth in, we could only think of doing this at a hotel which was right across the street from the hospital, and of course, part of a Birth Plan is to have a backup plan of using the hospital; natural and without drugs.

There were bumps in the pregnancy that caused some stress! For both of us, and, looking back with an eye open to the thyroid issues, I remember meeting with Dr. Mary Kirk, in San Jose, who was my OB/GYN and relating, that I had no breast changes? I asked repeatedly, as I had no bottles and had no intention of using "*formula*" ever. I was repeatedly told that everybody can **breast feed**, and, not to worry!

Radiation affects your glands and your **mammary gland tissue** can also be affected as well as your development as I have stated in this book. I had no breast changes because I lacked sufficient mammary gland tissue. Many women like myself were also told we had **dense breast tissue** upon review of a mammogram. Thyroid gland imbalances as a child can create a lot of havoc with your life and another reason I wrote this book is because I want others I care about to have the information when they are ready to hear it.

One of the things you can find written about thyroid gland imbalances is the issues of **giantism** (being very tall and even as far as Marfan syndrome), as well as **dwarfism**. I had no clue about that back then. I was somewhere about 20 weeks pregnant with my son, and I was asked by my

Doctor to go to another ultrasound at Stanford University for a follow up ultrasound. Following that appointment, I learned that it was to rule out **dwarfism** with my son, by remeasuring his limbs; I was beside myself that this was even a possibility; how could this happen? I mean when your doctor sends you to Stanford University you know something is serious! I was terribly stressed and worried.

At my next regularly scheduled OB visit, Dr. Kirk warned me against my diet which was vegetarian, high raw, and the possibility of neural tube defects. After the Stanford scare and later learning it was to rule out dwarfism, I complied with the request to begin eating other "protein" sources of which I would agree, like tuna and eggs. I have felt great, vibrant, full of energy and was walking a minimum of 3 miles per day and still going to African dance class while pregnant, joyful and happy.

Not only was this dietary change, really out of character for me and my belief about my body and how it fared the best but I did not feel too good eating these things. Our Midwife failed on us, relating she was exposed to spinal meningitis, and so we used our backup plan and my son was born in the hospital a *natural* vaginal birth 8 pounds with a 9/9 apgar. While he "latched on," and I produced the colostrum, many days later at home, I learned I was not producing nearly enough **breastmilk** and he cried, arched his back and, I did my best to comfort him. I made phone calls to the nurse back in San Jose from the new place I was renting in Santa Cruz having moved a month before birth, and she assured me it was colic.

My son cried more and more, his father was there but we were unsure of what to do, he was just a little guy 6 days old I just felt something was wrong. As a first time Mom, under the stress of feeling instinctively he was not getting enough to sustain him, I contacted my insurance company quickly and verified I could bring my son to Dominican Hospital in Santa Cruz. I trusted my intuition thankfully despite being told it was likely colic and his father getting upset that I was spoiling him, and we went to the emergency room with a slightly dehydrated infant, and, we ended up waiting. My son was days old, dehydrated and crying as he was hungry and I had no bottles and nobody around me really to jump in and help out, I had no idea what to do which is why I highly encourage support systems for moms and dads; for everyone.

The staff at the hospital left us in a room for far too long and my son being dehydrated began to show signs of escalating jaundice he was becoming quite orange and an attendant after trying to do a blood test on a 6 day old infant with dehydration unsuccessfully despite my repeatedly saying he was dehydrated eft the room for quite some time until the door opened finally and we were walked to the Neo-Natal Intensive Care Unit Level II and the nurses were waiting by the NICU incubator. They tried to get an IV into him in various ways but it would not take and by the 9th time, I had dropped to the floor silently begging for his life, on the 10th try, the IV took in his head.

I was asked to go upstairs to a room prepared for me and get some rest but I would not leave his side where he was in the incubator-the jaundice lights on him to bring down the jaundice. I sat by him and whispered "I love you so much Zahwa and I want you here!" I also now realize having looked at his baby pictures as I have asked you to do as well with your family that he was hypothyroid due to my maternal iodine deficit, stress, and dehydration at 6 days of age. I look back at his pictures and remember my friend asking me about his face. Of course as a new mother, your baby is absolutely perfect, I now see where he had edema in his facial tissues for sure. That was brought back under control in months and then at puberty I see pictures after moving to Minnesota where the shiners came under his eyes and stress of puberty and other factors brought him back into severe hypothyroidism. I believe at this time it may be autoimmune considering he began with horrid migraines by age 7. Looking back at those pictures will give you a lot of clues. Puffy face, swollen eyes, dark shiners, eating wheat and cheese and lots of dairy, school lunches and this could be the launch into ADHD or ODD if you can see this in the way that I do. It was a very stressful time and he lost a chunk of his precious childhood because we did not know as we both lost it.

Today, one of our benefits is having the internet and all the threads, are that we are able to bounce something off of somebody else and ask— but then, I did not have that.

To have the ability to jump on and ask questions with other women or get a recipe for making my own formula for my son. It was only a few months later and my son was super healthy and thriving. It was 1996 and I was making a formula from cooked squash, hemp seeds and alternative milks that I had enjoyed especially after reading the ingredients on the formula cans, I realize just about anything was better than that stuff! I wanted to know what was so special about the ingredients in formula and realized I could do better. I absolutely could not breast feed no matter what, not fennugreek, not acupuncture and human placenta tea in 1995, nor anything else I tried, I lacked the mammary gland tissue and was had **Hypoplasiainsufficient glandular tissue**.

I ended up making my own **formula, in 1996** which was healthful and several combinations of delicious blended drinks that I put into a bottle for my son and since I could not breast feed, I found that these greatly enhanced his nutrition.

When your children are young you have control over what they eat and it is the time to set down a good foundation so children will return to it even if they veer from it for some time the seeds will be planted. For my son from birth to age 6 nearly 7 when we moved to Minnesota just about everything he ate was organic and nearly all vegetarian. He was vibrant and a beacon of health, his intelligence and drive to learn were very high, and he was kind and playful. He absolutely loved going to school and he wanted challenges to learn. He and I would go get a burrito at Jalapeño's in Santa Cruz and from the time I could sit him on the counter as he watched them cut and chop and prepare fresh foods that we would take the beach and eat together to the Wednesday Farmer's Markets where we both got fresh cold pomegranate juice, his nutrition which was rich with minerals really took good care of him.

I had the experience of both, this way of life and what happened when he began eating the school lunches once we relocated to Minnesota and he formed dark circles under his eyes at about age 9 and just as puberty was beginning to come in I began to see major changes. His thyroid was stressed, nutritionally depleted and I now can reflect upon a long standing hypothyroid that was left without mineral help and it cost us both dearly.

Moving to Minnesota into a Goiter Belt we had a lot to adapt to, lack of sunlight, iodine, selenium, stress, and a poor school lunch system, all contributed. While the slower pace and the beautiful and abundant nature were positive it is a small city known for major and toxic pollution coming from factories with a paper mill nearby, brought more thyroid issues.

I asked for medical testing on two occasions and I was found to be in the normal range for thyroid issues and I ended up with a stressful situation in 2008 involving my son which caused me to end up in the hospital where I ended up with 3 different diagnosis. Stress based colitis, C. Diff and Ovarian Carcinoma. My CA125 was elevated over triple and my gut was stressed. I was told to come back for a surgery as soon as possible for a complete hysterectomy but I waited over a year and some months and handled it myself watching my test scores come down progressively. I have learned a great deal and felt more comfort, trust and ease in listening to my heart and mind about figuring out what I needed to do to heal.

Signs are often dismissed that would save somebody a lot of grief. We need to ask real questions about why we have so much radiation in our atmosphere? Why we allow so many of the foods that most people purchase and consume, as well as soft drinks. We have so many people who are obese, and suffering from issues, most of which could be prevented but we keep selling products and we keep selling responses to the problems? Why not strengthen the whole and begin to shift how we see what is happening and regenerate people versus sell them the same familiar and predictable food and medical industry responses. There are so many ways we can tell if somebody is degenerating and they are not well. We medicate everything and we do not know what we do. Placing IUDs and birth control sticks, pills and yet more hormones into our bodies is asking for disaster.

I hope that this book is helpful to you in the same way that you too can heal yourself.

It is not only our people suffering from thyroid imbalances but also the dogs I meet at the dog park, and just today my cousin Nancy brought by some fresh produce from her beautiful farm and she related about the **baby calves and how today they receive an injection of selenium on their first day or life**. When I asked her is she knew why this was happening today she said that **otherwise they will have a large thick tongue and they could die**. It was the perfect opportunity to introduce her to my work helping people reverse disease and heal and to tell her about this book about thyroid issues. Thyroid issues have always been much steeper in Northern Minnesota because it has low selenium and iodine. Our soils are vastly depleted from the way we produce food today and the halogens in the irrigation water. There are a few people who have well water that is clean and plentiful and have farmed their land for many years that will have clean food but the people have temporarily lost their way and the animals suffer.

# APPENDIX - RECIPES

### Sea Veggie Broth

6 cups distilled or filtered water
  4 large pieces of nori, DULSE or WAKAME
  1 tablespoon grape seed oil
  2 celery stalks and leaves, chopped
  1" piece of ginger root peeled and chopped
  1 carrot thinly sliced
  4 green stick onions, chopped
  1 pound of crimini mushrooms sliced
  Start with sea veggies and water over medium, add in the veggies,
a bit of salt, perhaps some
  Onion and garlic powder, and a bit of iodized sea salt. Cook on
medium or very gently as you
  Desire and serve warm.

### Detox & Heal Me Herbal Tea

2 Tablespoons dried nettle leaf
  2 Tablespoons dried alfalfa leaf
  2 Tablespoons red clover flowers
  1 Tablespoon oat straw
  1 Tablespoon dandelion root
  2 Tablespoons dried mint

Boil your water and pour over herbs in a French press or other
steeping pot for herbs, allow to

Infuse into the warm water for at least 15 minutes or more, and enjoy!

**Blue Vervain & Lavender**

1/2 teaspoon blue vervain leaf
1/2 teaspoon lavender flowers
1 large mug of hot water

Pour your hot water into your French press or pot to steep herbs over the vervain and lavender
Sweeten, and enjoy!

# ABOUT THE AUTHOR

Karen is real, present and authentic: that makes people love her, or it makes them very uncomfortable. You must be able to distinguish today between all the hype and the real truth.

She has been gathering Original Medicine for decades, including raw foods and cancer, juicing, detoxification are among many from early on. A Plant-Based Nutritionist, Herbalist, Massage Therapist, Certified Kemetic Yoga Teacher, Worked at the Santa Cruz Waldorf School, learned NVC Language, Cross-Cultural Communication, African dance and African Hand Drumming. She feels communication is very important.

Original Medicine, rarely seen today practiced by Elders, is something quite different from the dominant Western Allopathic Medicine today. We often think of medicine as one particular lane or specialization, yet Original Medicine people, and, there are very few remaining, may have as in Karen's case, many decades of Mind Body Medicine (Psychosomatics) and the use of a very uncommon intuitive ability. Everything is common sense as she has watched the "studies" and theories come and go.

Our interconnection with Nature, sensing through *The Field* and Nature's playful expression, the animals, birds, butterflies and the ways that we sense that are not just tangible and empirical, measured and factual, but they are nonetheless, valuable, insightful and revealing. They are a way that is taught very seldom today, as compared to entering the office to relate our symptoms.

A walk with a Shaman in Nature would be to observe your footing, your mind, your clarity, and what presents on your walk together is restorative, and provides opportunity for observation and real growth. Nature is a profound healer.

As a young girl, she spent many years learning the "old ways," and learning to use her mind, learning about perception. Her mother said something that really stuck with her when she was quite young: *"**What the Mind Perceives the Mind Believes**."*

She has given extensive insights perceptively and intuitively much differently than a diagnosis from a Western Doctor, she relates by sensing the body and The Field quite accurately. Clients over the years were shocked when she felt what they were feeling just before they arrived for appointments as energy is felt, and often our connections are symbiotic. Learning from the years of giving reflexology she can ascertain issues with internal organs and calcifications present in the form of stones, blockages and other issues on many levels-body mind and spirit is not just a common phrase but her everyday life and how she senses.

A Certified Family Law Specialist Paralegal for nearly 18 years, in private firms, the courts and the District Attorney, she developed strong research skills that enabled her to read and study quickly and speak professionally.

She enjoys public speaking and has given numerous workshops, courses and presentations. She thrives best, getting out and into Nature, meeting people, travel, spending time with the dogs, and, at the dog parks, yoga, and of course, reading. Coconut water, tropical fruits, and people who wish to gift something positive and real for the world! She loves life!

CPSIA information can be obtained
at www.ICGtesting.com
Printed in the USA
LVHW041123230320
650895LV00008B/2495